GW00382311

Perinatal Nursing

RECENT ADVANCES IN NURSING

Already published

Current Issues in Nursing
Edited by Lisbeth Hockey

Care of the Aging
Edited by Laurel Archer Copp

Cancer Nursing
Edited by Margaret C. Cahoon

Nursing Education
Edited by Margaret Steed Henderson

Primary Care Nursing
Edited by Lisbeth Hockey

Patient Teaching
Edited by Jenifer Wilson-Barnett

Communication
Edited by Ann Faulkner

Forthcoming Titles in the Series

Maternal and Infant Health
Edited by Mary Houston

Measuring the Quality of Care
Edited by Lucy D. Willis and Marjorie E. Linwood

Psychiatric Nursing
Edited by A.T. Altschul

Pain
Edited by Laurel Archer Copp

Long-Term Care
Edited by Kathleen King

Research Methodology
Edited by Margaret C. Cahoon

Clinical Nursing Practice
Edited by Alison J. Tierney

VOLUME EDITOR

Peggy-Anne Field RN SCM PhD FRSA

Peggy-Anne Field was trained as a nurse and midwife, and worked as a midwife in the United Kingdom before moving to Canada in 1957. She was a staff nurse, head nurse and instructor in maternal-newborn nursing at the Royal Victoria Hospital, Montreal, for 7 years. In 1964, following a period at McGill University, Montreal, she moved to the University of Alberta, Edmonton, as instructor in the Advanced Obstetrics Program. She has been consulted on nursing education programs in maternal-newborn care across Canada. She has been published widely in the areas of qualitative research and on various aspects of maternal-newborn care. In 1973–74 she spent a sabbatical year in England working as a staff-midwife for 6 months and studying delivery care in the community for the remaining time. She is a founder of the Western Nurse Midwives Association, Canada. Her current position is that of Professor of Nursing, teaching in both undergraduate and graduate programs at the University of Alberta.

EDITORIAL BOARD

Margaret C. Cahoon RN PhD

Dr Cahoon is Rosenstadt Professor of Health Research at the School of Nursing, University of Toronto, Canada. She has wide experience as a teacher, adviser and author. She is a former Fellow of the World Health Organization and a past president of the Ontario Public Health Association. At present she is the principal investigator in the Sunnybrook-University of Toronto Project for the development of a collaborative nursing research demonstration unit. She has made important contributions through her work in community health and oncology; she has been involved in studies of patient care and coping.

Laurel Archer Copp RN PhD FAAN

As Dean and Professor at the School of Nursing, University of North Carolina at Chapel Hill and a Fellow of the American Academy of Nursing, Dr Copp is an established nursing authority, having contributed over 60 articles to international nursing journals, instigated ten research studies and served on a number of important advisory committees. Her main interest is the psychology and philosophy of pain and suffering but her studies have ranged widely to investigate many aspects of research and the nursing curriculum. Her current appointments include Chairman of the Alumni Council of the Harvard Program on Health System Management and Chairman of the Task Force on Research of the American Association of Colleges of Nursing.

Lisbeth Hockey OBE FRCN Hon FRCGP SRN HV QNS PhD

Dr Hockey, a Fellow of the Royal College of Nursing, is well known as the Director of the First Nursing Research Unit established in the U.K. at the Department of Nursing Studies, Edinburgh University, in 1971, a post which she held from 1971–82. After practical experience as a district nurse, midwife and health visitor she specialised in teaching, administration and, above all, research. She developed a Research Department at the (then) Queen's Institute of District Nursing, undertaking and guiding research in community nursing. Her post in Edinburgh involved her in research in the wider field of nursing. She is currently a member of several national committees and past Chairman of the Royal College of Nursing Research Society.

RECENT ADVANCES IN NURSING 8

Perinatal Nursing

Edited by

Peggy-Anne Field
RN SCM PhD FRSA
Professor, Faculty of Nursing, The University of
Alberta, Edmonton, Alberta, Canada

Foreword by

Miss A.S. Grant
OBE RGN SCM MTD
Formerly Education Officer, Central Midwives Board for
Scotland

CHURCHILL LIVINGSTONE
EDINBURGH LONDON MELBOURNE AND NEW YORK 1984

CHURCHILL LIVINGSTONE
Medical Division of Longman Group Limited

Distributed in the United States of America by
Churchill Livingstone Inc., 1560 Broadway, New York,
N.Y. 10036, and by associated companies, branches
and representatives throughout the world.

© Longman Group Limited 1984

All rights reserved. No part of this publication
may be reproduced, stored in a retrieval system,
or transmitted in any form or by any means,
electronic, mechanical, photocopying, recording
or otherwise, without the prior permission of the
publishers (Churchill Livingstone, Robert Stevenson
House, 1–3 Baxter's Place, Leith Walk,
Edinburgh EH1 3AF).

First published 1984

ISBN   0 443 02811 7
ISSN   0144–6592

British Library Cataloguing in Publication Data
Perinatal nursing. — (Recent advances in nursing,
   ISSN 0144–6592)
   1. Obstetrics   2. Obstetrical nursing
   3. Infants (Newborn) — Care and hygiene
   I. Field, Peggy-Anne   II. Series
   618.3'2'0024613   RG524

Library of Congress Cataloging in Publication Data
Perinatal nursing.
   (Recent advances in nursing, ISSN 0144–6592;   )
   Bibliography: p.
   Includes index.
   1. Obstetrical nursing.   2. Pregnancy, Complications
of — Nursing.   3. Infants (Newborn) — Diseases — Nursing.
   I. Field, Peggy-Anne.   II. Series [DNLM:
   1. Obstetrical nursing.   2. Perinatology — Nursing texts.
   W1 RE105VN v. 8 / WY 157 P445]
   RG951.P57   1984   610.73'678   83–6634

Printed in Singapore by Selector Printing Co (Pte) Ltd

Foreword

During the past 20–30 years the quality of maternal and fetal life has been improved by a great upsurge in knowledge and by many technological advances. Childbirth today is safer than ever before. This achievement is recognised with satisfaction and gratitude. It has coincided, however, with an increasing complexity of ethical problems and scientific procedures and, most importantly, with the expanding and exploding expectations of the recipients of the service. All these changes make it imperative that attention is directed to skills in communication and that consideration is given to conceptual and perceptual abilities in counselling.

The nurse/midwife requires to assume new responsibilities and she is increasingly called upon to give intelligent and informed replies to questions on current issues. At one time some of these issues might have been considered as outwith the province of the nurse/midwife. This is no longer so. The total needs of the pregnant woman, her family and her environment have to be dealt with effectively and compassionately. The nurse/midwife should be aware of the implications of ethical issues in reproduction, of the independent judgement required for decision-making and of the changes in attitudes of society to the childbearing process. It is timely, therefore, that a book highlighting issues in perinatal nursing has been compiled.

Teamwork is central to the provision of a high standard of care; the successful outcome of many 'high-risk' pregnancies depends on a team approach. The team approach has been exemplified in the preparation of this book, with contributions coming from Australia, Canada, Sweden, the United Kingdom and the United States. Professor Peggy-Anne Field is to be congratulated on the selection of material which indicates sound judgement and a sense of balance. The contributors have brought the resources of their wide experience to the problems of today. Emphasis on concern and caring permeates each chapter.

It is my hope that the book will stimulate discussion and encourage nurse/midwives to acquire advanced knowledge in understanding of physiology and treatment. A fresh, cool look is necessary at certain aspects of the management of pregnancy, labour and the postnatal period and of the low birthweight infant. It is necessary to question long-cherished beliefs and to initiate research on midwifery practice. Solutions should be based on objective fact. The extensive reading list for more detailed study is welcomed and will prove of immense value in the continuing education of nurse/midwives. I wish the book every success, confident that it will prove intellectually stimulating and professionally rewarding.

Edinburgh 1984   Annie S. Grant

Preface

The field of perinatal nursing is very broad, encompassing prenatal, intrapartal and postpartum phases of care. While the term perinatal is generally taken to mean care of mothers and newborn at risk, the debate relating to maternal-newborn care continues as to whether or not all women need to be treated as if they were potentially at risk. Parents' rights, and the ethical issues associated with consumers' rights to information and input into their own care, are a critical part of today's debates on perinatal care. It is also my belief that nurses and midwives must understand physiological concepts and principles of medical management in order to provide appropriate nursing care. It was with these factors in mind that the content for this book was selected.

The first two chapters address the issues of the ethics related to reproduction and the place of birth. The following chapter examines the medical management and nursing care of parents in the prenatal period. Some current practices in labour and the relationship between parental desires and safe practice are then examined. One treatment that parents are questioning is the use of eye prophylaxis, and research related to the use of silver-nitrate is presented so that nurses may better answer parents' questions. The next two chapters present research on the physical care of the low birthweight infant and parents' reactions to prematurity, with the implications for nursing care resulting from the study findings. The final chapter presents recent research on postpartum depression, an area of nursing that has been too long ignored.

The annotated bibliography is designed to provide nurses with background information on selected topics as well as content related to relevant nursing actions. Genetic counselling is a relatively new field for nursing, so the authors were chosen with the aim of providing the nurse with an overview of the genetic counselling field, as well as with an evaluation of the effectiveness of existing programs.

The section on sexually transmitted diseases was selected with the community health nurse, school nurse and occupational health nurse in mind. The articles were also chosen so as to provide an international perspective whenever possible.

The editor would like to thank Miss Annie Grant, OBE, formerly Education Officer to the Central Midwives Board for Scotland, for providing the Foreword.

The work of individual authors in this book is to be commended. Several are experienced authors who are already internationally known, but for some it is their first effort at sharing their knowledge through publication. Their willingness to write for this volume cannot but help contribute to the future development of perinatal nursing.

Edmonton 1984   Peggy-Anne Field

Contributors

Dyanne D. Affonso RN PhD
Associate Professor, Division Coordinator, Psychiatric and Mental Health Nursing, University of Arizona, USA

Anita B. Bennetts RN CNM DrPH
Chief Nurse Manager of Field Services, Office of Community Health Services, Oregon State Health Division, Portland, Oregon, USA

Patricia M. Coward RN BN MN
Director of Nursing, Pediatric Pavilion, Royal Alexandra Hospital, Edmonton, Alberta, Canada

Peggy-Anne Field RN SCM PhD
Professor, Faculty of Nursing, The University of Alberta, Edmonton, Alberta, Canada

J.V. Lissenden SRN SCM
Sister, Royal Women's Hospital, Melbourne, Victoria, Australia

M.L. Romney SRN SCM
Research Sister, Division of Midwifery and Pediatrics, Northwick Park Hospital, Harrow, UK

Janet L. Storch RN BScN MHSA
Associate Professor, Department of Health Services Administration and Community Medicine, The University of Alberta, Edmonton, Alberta, Canada

Vivian Wahlberg RN RM BA DMedSc
Researcher and University Lecturer, Karolinka Institute, Stockholm, Sweden

V.G.L. White SRN SCM
Director of Nursing Services, Midwifery and Pediatrics, Northwick Park Hospital, Harrow, UK

Contents

PART ONE

Ethical issues in reproduction

INTRODUCTION

Among the more controversial ethical issues in health care today are those relating to the care surrounding human reproduction. This is so because a hierarchy of human values circumscribe the relationships and institutions regulating reproductive behavior (Report, 1981). Questions about the rightness or wrongness of medical interventions in the processes of human reproduction confront clinicians, patients, scientists, and society.

Dramatic medical-technical advances have occurred in health care, and nowhere so remarkedly as in reproductive technology. New discoveries have resulted in new abilities for medical science to intervene in procreative practices, from genetic interventions to interventions in the neonatal period. These advances have set the stage for a conflict of values.

Further, the decision to bear or not to bear a child is a profoundly personal and significant decision for the individual involved. Women have deep feelings about their reproductive capacity, and about having choices in relation to that capacity.

The issues at stake in answering the questions of right and wrong involve the extent of the freedom granted to individuals to make personal decisions regarding reproduction, the reasons for these decisions, and the consequences of the decisions for society as a whole. Because so many of these decisions challenge traditional values, rational approaches in responding to the questions are critical.

In this chapter, the range and variety of ethical issues involved in human reproduction will be discussed. While issues relating to contraception, sterilization and abortion may not seem to fit into issues of perinatal care, they are included here for two reasons. First, they represent historical and/or future problems for many individuals in perinatal care. Second, they so clearly demonstrate the strongly held societal beliefs and values associated with human reproduction and perinatal practices.

Ethical issues which arise from the control of genetic quality, and the control of the processes of procreation through artificial means are also included here as critical newer dimensions of perinatal care. Finally, attention is directed toward ethical issues of prenatal care, labor and delivery, and postnatal care, including care of the neonate.

DECISIONS NOT TO BEAR CHILDREN

The practices of contraception, sterilization, and abortion allow individuals to decide not to bear children. Each of these practices have been the focus of ethical conflict, either in an historical context or in current practice.

Contraception

As mortality rates declined in the Western world, it became feasible to entertain thoughts of population control by means of contraceptive practice. Late in the 18th century, Thomas Malthus warned that population growth would outstrip the capacity to feed humanity and his warnings seem to have been one factor in precipitating moves towards the birth control campaigns of the 19th century (Fromer, 1981). In the United States there followed many attempts to make birth control illegal, including the Comstock law of 1873. It was not until the late 1930s, however, following arrests and convictions of one, Margaret Sanger, who established birth control information clinics and worked to disseminate birth control literature, that the laws were finally relaxed (Reich, 1978). But even as late as 1965, Planned Parenthood personnel in Connecticut were arrested and convicted. The outcome of this final conviction was the reversal of the decision by the U.S. Supreme Court and the apparent confirmation of a constitutional right to privacy in contraceptive decision-making (Wing, 1976). These examples are indicative of the deeply held beliefs that it was considered wrong to interfere in acts of nature. Such interference challenged traditional values and beliefs, and led to considerable ethical debate.

Today, the central ethical issues in contraception center on two main issues: (1) the rightness or wrongness of prescribing contraceptives for minors, and (2) the individual's access to sufficient information about various means of contraception. Except for those who hold certain religious beliefs, the acceptability of contraception is relatively widespread. However, there is considerable ambiguity in determining if minors can also have access to contraception, where there is an overriding concern about sexual permissiveness. The ethics of withholding such information from individuals who are sexually active must be examined. Does a minor have to prove sexual activity by bearing a child or applying for abortion, to receive contraceptive teaching and prescription?

There is concern too that women do not always have the information they need to make choices regarding contraception; that intramuscular hormones (such as Depo-Provera) and intrauterine devices (such as the Dalkon Shield), are or have been prescribed for women who do not understand their true effects and risks (Fromer, 1981; Savage, 1982). This is particularly true in respect to marketing these products in Third World nations.

Sterilization

There has been a cautious approach to sterilization for purely contraceptive purposes. Under English law, the Offences Against Person Act of 1861, while not expressly forbidding sterilization, resulted in an avoidance of the issue of sterilization by most physicians. As recently as 1954 an English judge voiced his concern about sex without responsibility, stating that sterilization surgery was 'injurious to the public interest...degrading to the man...and injurious to the wife.' (Kouri, 1976).

Although public attitudes and values have changed over the past 30 years, there are a number of ethical-legal issues surrounding sterilization which remain. A major issue concerns the adequacy of information provided to the candidate for sterilization. Is it sufficient information to enable an informed decision and consent? The increasing requests for reversals of the sterilization process, and the apparent regional variations in the numbers of sterilizations, raise concern that full alternatives may not have been adequately presented to those seeking contraceptive assistance (Savage, 1982).

A second issue concerns the legal cases of wrongful birth and wrongful life which have arisen following failed sterilizations. These cases challenge basic values. In wrongful birth the plaintiff (the parent or parents) brings an action against the defendant (usually a physician) charging that because of his negligence, the birth of a child occurred causing injury for which damages should be awarded

(Robertson, 1978)*. The majority of judges in the recorded cases have stated that it is against public policy to award damages for the birth of a child. In other words the judges have assessed that the majority of citizens would value a respect for a newly born infant, which does not allow a claim for damages because that infant has been born.

A third issue concerns the sterilization of the mentally retarded. Out of a fear of perceived eugenic manipulation, many countries have moved towards restrictions in access to sterilization for the mentally retarded, in order to protect their rights. Yet, some of these restrictions work against those who could benefit from the protection sterilization can offer. The ethical dilemma of providing protection against undesired sterilization for the mentally retarded while trying to enable sterilization when it seems in the best interests of the retarded child or adult, is a complex problem (Report, 1979).

Abortion

Abortion is one of the most controversial issues, particularly in North American society. It is viewed by some as the 'battle-ground for reproductive rights' and 'a crucible in which to test the nation's morality' (Churchill & Simán, 1982). In the U.S., a number of legal cases have drawn attention to these value disputes, and there has been much activity at Senatorial level to restrict access to abortions, and to make abortion illegal (Campbell, 1978). In Canada there has been less public furor but the same value conflicts prevail. Abortion law is applied in a highly erratic manner with considerable disparity in access to abortion services. The Mortgentaler trials in Quebec highlighted the discrepancies in Canadian abortion law and the uncertainties of the dilemma (Dickens, 1976; Report, 1977).

The ethical issues in abortion seem to involve three main foci: the status of the fetus, the problems of conflicting claims, and the consequences for society as a whole. There are many conflicting values regarding the status of the fetus as a human being. Some hold that at conception the human being is formed; others argue that the status of being a human being occurs at implantation, or when the fetus 'looks like' a human, or at 'quickening', or at the point it would

---

*Wrongful life is a term to denote similar action brought by the child against a physician, pharmacist, or clinical laboratories. Apart from cases of wrongful birth and wrongful life in failed sterilization, actions have also been brought to court regarding improper dispensing of a contraceptive failed abortion, and incorrect laboratory results in prenatal diagnosis.

be viable outside the mother's womb, or simply, when it is born. These decisions are not based in factual knowledge as much as in cherished values about when life begins (Bok, 1974). And no resolution of these issues appears forthcoming. Some suggest that the concept of personhood as distinct from human being might assist in clarifying the issues.

The problem of conflicting rights is related to the debate about the status of the fetus. Whose rights are foremost — the rights of the fetus or the rights of the mother? Judith Thomson (1971) argues that the fetus is a person for whom a woman has a special responsibility, particularly when she has assumed that responsibility implicitly or explicitly, and that abortion should not be impermissible, but neither should it always be permissible. Other authors object to the use of rights claims, and to the suggestion that valuing fetal life always should transcend the needs of others in decisions. They argue that fetal life should be valued and protected, but so should newborn, adolescent, and adult life be protected; greater responsibility must be accepted for the quality of life of persons already born (Churchill & Simán, 1982).

The consequences of abortion for society as a whole must also be considered. Since all society has a stake in protecting life, care must be taken to clarify the justifications for abortion so that some guidelines might be agreed upon. This is the 'thin edge of the wedge' argument, that is, that we may become so liberal in our values that newborn infants may be included in legal killing (Bok, 1974).

DECISIONS ABOUT GENETIC QUALITY

Advances in medical technology have profoundly affected the ability to detect hereditary disease in the prenatal period. Down's syndrome and neural tube defects are two of the most common genetic defects detectable in early pregnancy. Methods of screening range from maternal serum examination to ultrasonography, fetoscopy and amniocentesis. In the main, these defects are only detectable, not treatable. (Exceptions occur, of course, in some beginning areas of fetal surgery, or where a fetus might be transfused while in the womb).

Because diagnosis can be made without recourse to treatment a number of ethical issues surface. Will the diagnosis be provided as information to couples in order to allow them to make decisions about terminating or maintaining a pregnancy? Or will couples feel coerced into termination should a genetic problem be detected? Joseph Fletcher, prominent theologian and moral philosopher in the United States, holds strong views on this matter. He has stated that it is unethical to 'knowingly and deliberately victimize' innocent others, and that to bring knowingly a diseased or defective child into the world injures society, the family, and the individual born (Hard Choices, 1981).

These views are counterbalanced by those individuals who believe in the autonomy, and therefore, freedom of choice for the parents including choices to choose abortion to terminate the pregnancy, to bring the child to term prepared for the condition, or to surrender the child for adoption following birth (Powledge & Fletcher, 1979).

There is, of course, the continuing question of who decides what is to be considered normal, a question of eugenics. As genetic technology expands, it is possible that smaller deviations from the norm will be detectable. How much or how little deviation might society eventually tolerate? Ethical questions have been raised, as well, in regard to decision-making if only one twin is affected. By Fletcher's standards, this would be a most difficult dilemma; the choice of sacrificing the normal fetus or giving birth to a defective child so a normal one might live. There is also the question of a late abortion. Due to delays in obtaining the results of an amniocentesis, a woman may elect to terminate the pregnancy by hysterotomy at a time when a viable fetus might result. What should be the fate of a live fetus in this instance? Other questions concern the appropriate use of amniocentesis. Since it is possible to determine the gender of the fetus, should parents be given this information and be allowed to abort for reasons of sex choice?

It seems clear that further genetic research is required to enable therapeutic intervention on the affected fetus following the diagnostic procedures. Prenatal diagnosis should be seen as a stop gap measure only. There is an equally urgent need to clarify values about normalcy, and about the acceptable limits to parental choice.

DECISIONS TO PROCREATE BY ARTIFICIAL MEANS

Two means of procreation by artificial means have the potential to change our reproductive habits. One means, artificial insemination by donor (AID), has been possible for some time; the other, in vitro fertilization (IVF), is a comparatively new technique. Widespread use of these techniques challenges our traditional understandings of the nature of sexuality, breeding, and the concept of parenthood

(Fromer, 1981; Report, 1981). How far will this technology lead us, that is, what are the consequences for society of the expansion of these technologies? What guidelines will be applied?

In terms of AID, some ethical quandaries relate to the selection of the donors, the potential for intermarriage of donors, problems of sperm-banking, the authority to conduct AID, and the deception now a part of AID. In Canada, the centres for AID are located within universities. There has been a tendency to recruit sperm donors from among students, particularly medical students. Such a practice is not uncommon, since medical students are convenient, generally reliable, and highly motivated individuals. This practice has led to charges that physicians are attempting to reproduce themselves — they are making eugenic choices (Annas, 1979). Elsewhere recruitment of sperm donors varies, but there can be a tendency to seek out highly intelligent individuals (for example, Nobel prize winners). The prevailing principle operative here may be that some people are more desirable than others. A related problem is the potential intermarriage of a single donor's offspring if the numbers of sperm donations are not controlled. There appears to be an urgent need to establish some guidelines in the best interest of society and future generations.

There are potential problems, too, in sperm banking and in the authority to conduct AID. In Canada, banking is largely restricted to the university centres, and the authority is considered to rest with a physician. Some have interpreted this move as a further attempt to 'medicalize' all of life. Yet, in the absence of guidelines or regulations, this may be a sensible approach, at least until these ethical concerns have been more carefully considered. There is a need to safeguard the practice of AID itself so it does not become perverse. Even with these safeguards in Canada, there are reported to be women's groups engaging in self-insemination practices, obtaining sperm via a physician's office. In the United States practices vary. In several states it is illegal for anyone other than a licensed physician to engage in AID, including self-insemination. In other areas, commercial sperm banks are preparing to market insemination kits directly to consumers' homes (Annas, 1979).

Sperm banking is problematic. Attention must be directed towards techniques of proper storage: yet there is insufficient knowledge to ensure that some sperm will not be damaged. Who will be responsible for children born defective as a result of damaged sperm?

A most serious ethical issue in AID is the problem of deception;

deception to the offspring and to society. Couples are often advised not to discuss AID with family or friends, and not to tell the offspring about his unique conception. There is the need, too, to protect the donors and their spouses from disclosure. When is it right to deceive? And is such deception in the best interests of the deceivers and the deceived?

The practice of in vitro fertilization raises another set of questions, albeit many related to AID. Because the manufacture of 'test-tube babies' (IVF products) involves the creation and frequently the destruction of human life, IVF practices have created ethical, legal, and medical controversy (Cohen, 1978). The unnaturalness of the procedure, the destruction of surplus embryos, the potential of damage to the embryo, and the whole question of resource allocation, are some of these questions.

There is an unnaturalness to this technique which may degrade parenthood and significantly alter mother-child relationships. It is possible that the development of this technique could result in sperm from one man being united with ovum from a woman which is fertilized and then implanted into the womb of a second woman who bears the child. Furthermore the child might then be raised by yet other individuals. IVF raises substantial questions about family relationships and child support (Strickland, 1981).

During the process of IVF, several ova may be extracted and fertilized to obtain the one chosen for implantation. The surplus embryos are then destroyed. As with the abortion issue, the question remains, what is the status of these embryos — are they human beings with rights?

Another concern relates to the newness of the technique. There is a potential for the embryo to be damaged during growth or re-insertion in the uterus. The risks are not only 'unknown but un-knowable' at this time. Is it ethical to subject an embryo to these hazards (Walters, 1979)?

In both AID and IVF the potential problems of surrogate mother-hood must be considered. What are reasonable limits to the use of surrogates? For example, if a career woman wishes to have a family, but does not wish the burden of a pregnancy, should she be permit-ted use of a surrogate? What if the surrogate failed to follow a healthy lifestyle in the prenatal period, could she be held liable for a defective or ill child? What about deception: what records should be kept of the arrangement? And how similar might these arrange-ments be to outright baby-selling?

The allocation of social resources is yet another issue in both AID and IVF. Does society agree that it is a basic right, at any expense, to have one's own children? Further, is resolution of infertility one of society's most pressing problems?

The social and ethical concerns related to AID and IVF require further consideration and thoughtful clarification of the central issues for individuals and society. With the development towards artificial placentas and artificial wombs, the concerns are serious and immediate. The technology cannot be allowed to direct society: society must guide the technology.

DECISIONS IN PRENATAL CARE, LABOR, AND DELIVERY

Birthing and preparation for birthing are generally regarded as highly significant events in a woman's (and her family's) life. During the past several decades there have been many changes in patterns of care in the perinatal period resulting in increased safety for mother and child, as evidenced by the decline in maternal and perinatal mortality rates. This has been accomplished by an increase in medical interventions in prenatal care, labor, and delivery (as well as in the care of the neonate). It is these interventions which have precipitated controversies in care, centering on the woman's right to autonomous decision-making in this special life event.

Ivan Illich (1975), a prominent social critic, has been most outspoken in his criticisms of the medical systems of the Western world for their medicalization of all of life. He draws attention to the expectations that women are to receive medical care during the prenatal period, challenging the medicalization of even this aspect of life. Although Illich's criticism has some merit, few would dispute the value of prenatal attention to prepare a woman for the birth experience, to detect early problems, and to ensure a more informed and capable mother. To this end, prospective mothers are urged to attend prenatal classes and to seek medical supervision during the pregnancy.

Some have argued, however, that the educational material and the formal classes for the prospective mother are often used to teach women how to conform to medical biases — they are taught to become more compliant and less independent (Katona, 1981; Oakley, 1982). This serves the needs of the health care system well, since it allows the health professionals to take charge, with limited participation by the woman in decision-making.

Another concern about much of prenatal education is the portrayal of an idealized image of birth. Too often the 'moment of birth' becomes the focus of education for childbirth while the events preceding and following are underemphasized. Women may therefore experience considerable frustration and disappointment if that 'moment' is not ideal. Emphasis on the nuclear family in the birthing event is also an ideal: a substantial number of women delivering babies today deliver alone (Katona, 1981; Laslie, 1982). There appears to be a great need for more balanced and realistic education, and for support in prenatal care.

Ethical issues in labor and delivery center on the respect accorded the mother by her involvement in making decisions during this event. The disputes about the role of the medical profession in the birthing process date back to at least the 1850s when there was controversy about the use of chloroform to relieve pain in childbirth. Ironically, the use of this pain-relieving agent was a challenge to obstetricians at that time. Queen Victoria's use and subsequent endorsement of chloroform in 1853 did little to dissuade the medical experts from arguing against its use. Later, 'natural childbirth,' as promoted by Grantly Dick-Read, also was seen as a threat (Katona, 1981). Today, the push toward home delivery has become the challenge to medical authority.

Anne Seiden (1978) has outlined three basic goals involved in assisting with the process of labor: (1) to enhance the safety of mother and child, (2) to allow freedom from unnecessary pain without dulling the senses to the positive aspects of the birth experience, and (3) to establish and maintain a good foundation for mother, child and family. There is concern that modern obstetrical practices concentrate on the first goal only — to enhance safety.

The home birth movement might be seen as a plea for recognition of other goals in childbirth, and a plea that physicians and hospitals be more responsive to the needs of their patients in labor and delivery (Laslie, 1982). There is a need to separate high risk mothers, who require highly technical services, from the normal birthing group, and to plan for birthing rooms and alternative birthing centers. None of these changes can be effective, however, unless accompanied by attitudinal changes on the part of the health professionals, and policy changes in the institutions providing care. Hospital maternity units, large and small, must review their policies to be sure they are humane and supportive to the family (Post, 1982). Further, the woman's right of informed choice must be respected.

In 1976, Valmai Elkins, Canadian childbirth educator, wrote a book entitled *The Rights of the Pregnant Parent*. In this book she discusses a number of obstetrical practices of concern to women: the need for information, the problem of positioning during labor and delivery, the use of oxytocic drugs to induce labor, the necessity of the shave preparation and enemata, the use of forceps in delivery and the practice of episiotomy. In a well-balanced presentation of these issues, she urges women to become more knowledgeable about these practices and to become more involved in decision-making regarding the interventions.

Presently there appears to be some ambivalence in allowing a woman in normal labor to control the situation: instead, choices are often removed from women and, in some cases, one intervention leads to another. Sometimes women in labor are accorded a child-like status and little is done to increase the woman's confidence, control and sense of mastery over the overall pregnancy and delivery (Laslie, 1982). There appears to be a need to balance the need to take advantage of the high technologies of obstetrical care as required, without being forced into undue interventions or being placed on the hospital's surgical agenda (Guillemin, 1981).

Electronic fetal monitoring (EFM) is a technology which was introduced into medical practice in the mid 1960s. As with many other new medical technologies, EFM was introduced without a satisfactory evaluation of its impact on morbidity and mortality (Banta & Thacker, 1979). EFM has been staunchly criticized on a number of grounds. First patients may not be well-informed of the minor risks in monitoring and they may not be given choices in use of the monitor. Second, monitoring may be used as a replacement of the physician's clinical judgement rather than as an adjunct to it. Third, reliance on monitoring may lead to misdiagnosis and un-necessary interventions. In answer to the critics, many obstetricians admit to problems of overreliance and over-utilization in the intro-duction of EFM, but contend that monitoring combined with clinic-al judgement (particularly in mothers at risk) results in early in-terventions which enhance the quality of the newborn.

One type of early intervention is the Caesarean section. Many feminist writers have been highly critical of intervention by Caesa-rean section. They point to the dramatic rise in Caesarean section rates across North America, England, Wales and Western Europe since the mid 1960s and often suggest a causal relationship between the introduction of EFM and increased sections. Although EFM may account for a small percentage of the increase, reasons of difficult labor, previous Caesarean section and breech presentation predominate (Bottoms et al, 1980; Wadhera & Nair, 1982).

A physician's reasons for choosing a surgical intervention are based on a greater understanding of the relationship between traumatic vaginal deliveries and neurological deficits, and between respiratory distress syndrome and neurological deficits; as well as the increased safety of the operation today compared to previous years. For many, there is a sense of relief that this option is now available to ensure a healthy baby. Yet the question of the necessity of this drastic intervention into a normal process continues to fester. Significant regional variations in rates fuel the controversy (Savage, 1982); and the percentage of sections done as repeat sections are worrisome, particularly since these are usually performed on young women destined to be repeaters (Wadhera & Nair, 1982). Is there any conflict of interest in choosing a Caesarean section? And, who should decide on the intervention?

DECISIONS IN NEONATAL CARE

The application of new knowledge in the care of the newborn resulted in a 58% decrease in the infant death rate in the United States between 1940 and 1970 (Duff & Campbell, 1973). Since, at least 1970, concern has extended 'beyond mere prevention of death to the question of the value of that life for which infants may now be saved.' (Jonsen, et al 1975).

When an infant is born healthy, the mother (and the father) generally desire consultation on the care of their newborn. They also want to be advised about potential problems of infant care, and want to be involved in making decisions about their resolution. By and large, these are not ethical decisions, but rather, matters of personal concern and preference.

Real ethical dilemmas are encountered, however, when decisions must be made about an infant who is not well, or who is seriously defective. Who decides whether the infant should be resuscitated and sustained, or whether aggressive efforts to prolong life should cease?

Many believe that this decision must rest with the parents since they are the 'true risk-takers and burden bearers' (Jonsen et al, 1975; Duff & Campbell, 1976). Others argue that parents may not be able to make a just decision, since they may not be able to 'consider adequately the independent rights of the infant as a unique individual.' (Abrams & Neumann, 1978). As an example of parental short-sightedness in decision-making, the much publicized case of the infant with Down's syndrome and duodenal atresia (at the Johns

Hopkins Hospital) is cited. In this case, the parents would not give their consent to life-preserving and correctable surgery, because the infant also had Down's syndrome (Duff & Campbell, 1973). Similar cases have been publicized across North America begging the question, who should decide?

Since it is extremely difficult to judge from a newborn's initial condition whether he will be ultimately healthy or defective, there appears to be a growing consensus that, barring severe abnormalities easily detectable at birth, infants should be resuscitated initially. This action provides a fairer opportunity to observe and assess the infant (Jonsen et al, 1975). Following initial assessment, parents should be given all the information so that they, with their professional advisers, can make a decision (Duff & Campbell, 1973). If it is not possible for families and attendant professionals to reach a mutual decision, an ethics committee may be called upon as an outside consulting body. Society should only intervene if three conditions are clearly present: (1) harm is being done to the infant, (2) a more suitable alternative is available, and (3) society is willing to support those on whom an unwelcome choice is imposed (Duff & Campbell, 1976).

IMPLICATIONS FOR NURSING

Identification of the ethical issues of human reproduction above serves to highlight the range and variety of ethical conflicts nurses encounter in perinatal nursing. The agony of supporting those making difficult choices is a very real stress for nurses in this area of health care. Common to most of the ethical issues discussed are the patients' (and families') need for information, support and freedom from coercion. Also necessary, in many of the conflicts, are guidelines for decision-making and structural changes to enable more supportive care. This means that nurses must be involved at two levels: the level of the individual patient, and at the level where policies and guidelines are developed.

Nurses and individual patients

Nursing has been described as a moral act; an art which involves both caring for and caring about patients and their families (Curtin & Flaherty, 1982). In human reproduction, families assume an increasingly important focus of the nurse's task. When nurses work with individuals or families who are deciding not to bear children (whether permanently or temporarily) they must be sensitive to the information needs: they must ensure that the individuals involved know the facts about the medication, device or surgery they are contemplating, and about alternatives available to them. In situations where abortion is the choice, nurses must ensure that their own religious or moral values are not imposed on the patient. Because it is difficult to provide good care in situations of moral conflict, a job transfer or change may be necessary to extricate the nurse from the conflict. As long as the patient's needs take precedence over the nurse's needs in, for example, emergency situations, a nurse's decision to remove herself from abortion care should be supported. Nurses who provide care to patients receiving abortions must be attentive to their needs for information, support, and confidentiality (Storch, 1982).

In assisting individuals and families involved in making decisions about genetic quality, the nurse's role in providing information and support is equally critical. Before genetic screening is commenced individuals need to know the nature and purpose of the screening, the potential consequences of screening, the risks of not undergoing the screening, and the possibility that inexact or inaccurate results may occur. Following general screening or prenatal diagnosis it is imperative that individuals be allowed the freedom to make their decision. Nurses must ensure that coercive counselling does not occur, and that alternatives are known by the patients. Patients confronted with test results which indicate a genetic problem need someone to listen to them and to assist them in understanding their choices (Storch, 1982). If their choice is to continue with the pregnancy, appropriate referrals should be made to provide support in both the prenatal and postnatal period.

Nurses caring for those who are choosing an artificial means of procreation, are involved on the frontiers of medical science. Although little guidance in these areas is yet available, two conditions should prevail. The individual needs to know as much as possible about the processes in which they are engaged, including the legal, moral and religious implications. Nurses can be instrumental in assessing the couple's level of understanding, in being available to listen and answer questions, and in supporting individuals through this value-laden event. Secondly, nurses must communicate a deep sense of respect and caring for these patients.

In caring for prenatal patients, and for individuals and families during childbirth, nurses have opportunities to educate and to support, in order to increase a woman's sense of self-mastery. As noted earlier, Seiden (1978) outlined goals of safety, freedom from unnecessary pain, and establishing a good foundation for mother, child and family, as important goals in childbirth. Safety has been given reasonable attention in both medical and nursing care, as has attention to freedom from unnecessary pain. But a goal not well attended to is the development of confidence and capability in the mother. Sometimes this goal may even conflict with the goals of safety and pain relief. Nurses must fill a sustaining role in this critical period of a family's life. Beginning in the prenatal period, teaching must be aimed at increasing the individual's self-reliance and confidence. This means that prospective mothers should be given sufficient information and be involved in decision-making. Teaching must be geared towards the importance of the whole process of childbearing, not just the few hours in labor or the moment of birth. These mothers also need an available, continuous contact person who can assist, encourage, and sustain, thus an apparent need for more nurse-midwives (Walker, 1976).

In the care of the neonate, parental decision-making must be supported. Nurses, while providing the best care possible for the infant, must support the parents who are ultimately responsible for the outcomes of any decision-making. If a difficult decision is made to discontinue treatment, nurses can be instrumental in ensuring that this will occur in the most humane way possible. Allowing the mother and family to hold the babe until death can enhance the family's process of grieving (Duff & Campbell, 1976). Or, the nurse may hold the infant until death.

Nurses and policies

Nurses must also be involved at the level where policies and guidelines are developed for the care and treatment of individuals and families in areas of human reproduction. In terms of abortion services, ways must be found to deal with this major social and moral problem. In the absence of adequate social support to the infants and children who are products of unwanted pregnancies, pious activities of pro-life groups are inadequate, unless they also are willing to support a quality of life for the children affected. Nurses must be involved in preventive efforts to decrease the need for abortion, and in developing policies allowing equitable access to care.

In two areas concerning human reproduction, genetic services, and in artificial insemination and in vitro fertilization services, there is an urgent need for guidelines. Some of these guidelines are in various stages of development: some are not yet begun. In genetic services, guidelines are essential for amniocentesis and other means of screening. Who should have access to these services? With what restrictions? Again, nurses must be involved in establishing reasonable and morally adequate guidelines. Of even greater urgency is the need for guidelines respecting AID and IVF, and possible future developments in related areas. Above all, abuse of these technologies must be prevented.

In prenatal care and in childbirth, nurses can be instrumental in supporting changes that will enhance goals of confidence in the mother, and a sense of control over her experience, while retaining due regard for goals of safety. This would involve a change in policies on maternity units which restrict family involvement, and which foster undue dependence. It also involves working towards attitudinal changes in all personnel, and changing structures to allow for maternal decision-making.

Finally, in the care of the defective or ill neonate, guidelines are necessary to allow for humane and responsible care. Nurses must be involved in instigating such guidelines (as necessary), and in formulating such a moral policy.

CONCLUSION

It is clear that the ethical issues in human reproduction are many — and for nurses, the challenges are great. Individuals and families have many advocacy needs: nurses have many opportunities to represent their patients. A fundamental need of these individuals is the need to be respected as decision-makers in care. Nurses have a significant role to fill in promoting this goal.

Acknowledgement

The author is indebted to the Alberta Educational Communications Corporation (ACCESS) for the opportunity to research this topic through their project on ethical issues in health care. This chapter and the ACCESS project paper were being developed simultaneously. The ACCESS project allowed resources for interviews to be conducted to substantiate, and enlarge on, the ethical issues identified in the literature.

REFERENCES

Abrams N, Neumann L L 1978 Human rights and ethical decision-making in the newborn nursery. In: Bandman B, Bandman E (eds) Bioethics and human rights. Little, Brown, Boston, p 159

Annas G J 1979 Artificial insemination: beyond the best interests of the donor. The Hastings Center 9: 14

Banta H, Thacker S B 1979 Policies toward medical technology: the case of electronic fetal monitoring. American Journal of Public Health 69: 931

Bok S 1974 Ethical problems of abortion. The Hastings Center 2: 33

Bottoms S F, Rosen M, Sokol R 1980 The increase in Caesarean birth rate. New England Journal of Medicine 302: 559

Campbell T 1978 Abortion law in Canada: a need for reform. Saskatchewan Law Review 42: 221

Churchill L, Simán J J 1982 Abortion and the rhetoric of individual rights. The Hastings Center 12: 9

Cohen M E 1978 The 'brave new baby' and the law: fashioning remedies for the victims of in vitro fertilization. American Journal of Law and Medicine 4: 319

Curtin L, Flaherty J 1982 Nursing ethics: theories and pragmatics. Robert J Brady, Bowie, Maryland

Dickens B M 1976 The Morgentaler case: criminal process and the abortion law. Osgoode Hall Law Journal 14: 229

Duff R S, Campbell A G M 1973 Moral and ethical dilemmas in the special-care nursery. New England Journal of Medicine 289: 890–894

Duff R S, Campbell A G M 1976 On deciding the care of the severely handicapped or drying persons: with particular reference to infants. Pediatrics 57: 487–493

Elkins V H 1976 The rights of the pregnant parent. Waxwing, Ottawa

Fromer M J 1981 Ethical issues in health care. C V Mosby, St Louis

Guillemin J 1981 Babies by Caesarean: who chooses, who controls? The Hastings Center 11: 15

Hard Choices 1981 Genetic screening. PTV Publications, Kent, Ohio

Illich I 1975 Medical nemesis. Calder and Boyars, London

Jonsen A R, Phibbs R H, Tooley W H, Garland M J 1975 Critical issues in newborn intensive care: a conference report and policy proposal. Pediatrics 55: 756–768

Katona C L E 1981 Approaches to antenatal education. Social Science and Medicine 15A: 25

Kouri R P 1976 The legality of purely contraceptive sterilization. Revue de droit 7: 1

Laslie A E 1982 Ethical issues in childbirth. The Journal of Medicine and Philosophy 7: 179

Oakley A 1982 The relevance of the history of medicine to an understanding of current change: some comments from the domain of antenatal care. Social Science and Medicine 16: 667

Post S 1982 Family centered care is a must. Hospital Trustee 6: 14

Powledge T M, Fletcher J 1979 Guidelines for the ethical, social and legal issues in prenatal diagnosis. New England Journal of Medicine 300: 168

Reich P 1978 A historical understanding of contraception. In: Notman M, Nadelson C (eds) The woman patient: medical and psychological interfaces. Plenum Press, New York

Report 1977 Report of the committee on the operation of the abortion law. Supply and Services, Ottawa

Report 1979 Sterilization: implications for mentally retarded and mentally ill persons. Law Reform Commission of Canada, Ottawa

Report 1981 Storage and utilization of human sperm. Health and Welfare Canada, Ottawa

Robertson G B 1978 Civil liability arising from 'wrongful birth' following an unsuccessful sterilization operation. American Journal of Law and Medicine 4: 131

Savage W 1982 Taking liberties with women: abortion, sterilization and
  contraception. International Journal of Health Services 12: 293
Seiden A M 1978 A sense of mastery in the childbirth experience. In: Notman M,
  Nadelson C The woman patient: medical and psychological interfaces. Plenum
  Press, New York
Storch J 1982 Patients' rights: ethical and legal issues in health care and nursing.
  McGraw-Hill Ryerson, Toronto
Strickland O L 1981 In vitro fertilization: dilemma or opportunity? Advances in
  Nursing Science 3: 41
Thomson J J 1971 A defense of abortion. Philosophy and Public Affairs 1: 47
Wadhera S, Nair C 1982 Trends in Caesarean section deliveries, Canada, 1968–1977.
  Canadian Journal of Public Health 73: 47
Walker J F 1976 Midwife or obstetric nurse? Some perceptions of midwives and
  obstetricians of the role of the midwife. Journal of Advanced Nursing 1: 129
Walters L 1979 Human in vitro fertilization: a review of the ethical literature. The
  Hastings Center 9: 23
Wing K R 1976 The law and the public's health. C V Mosby, St Louis

Freestanding birth centers

INTRODUCTION

This chapter will define the concept of the freestanding birth center (FBC), review its historical development and evaluate its role now and for the future. An understanding of the context in which these centers were created is essential for an appreciation of their influence on and contribution to maternity care today. Finally, although only limited data are available concerning the safety and satisfaction associated with FBC care, the United States FBC experience to date is reviewed.

DEFINITION

Birth centers exist in many countries throughout the world. However, in the United States these centers are a relatively recent phenomena. 99 FBCs are known to be providing maternity services in the U.S.A. as of December 1982 (Ernst, 1982). The majority of these centers offer certified nurse-midwifery care and are located on the periphery of the U.S.A. excluding the central portion of the country.

A freestanding birth center has been defined in a variety of ways depending on the author. However, for the purpose of licensure, the Cooperative Birth Center Network, a program of the Maternity Center Association (MCA) of New York, has defined it as follows:

A birth center is an adaptation of a home environment to a short stay, ambulatory, health care facility with access to in-hospital obstetrical and newborn services; designed to safely accommodate participating family members and support people of the woman's choice; and providing professional preventive health care to women and the fetus or newborn during pregnancy, birth and the puerperium. Any out-of-hospital setting where three or more births occur within one calendar year which is not a laboring woman's legal residence shall be defined as a birth center...

The professional group of practitioners responsible for the management of care of women and childbearing families in birth centers may represent one of the following collaborative arrangements: 1) Nurse-Midwifery: At least one certified nurse-midwife working in collaboration with a consulting physician who, if not a practicing obstetrician or surgeon, will have an agreement for consultation and referral with a practicing obstetrician or surgeon; 2) Family practitioner: At least one general physician with training in midwifery or obstetrics, appropriate professional; or 3) Obstetrician: At least one obstetrician with appropriate nursing and/or midwifery staff. All professional practitioners will limit their practice while caring for women during labor and birth in the birth center to the standards recommended by the American College of Nurse-Midwives and other appropriate national standard organizations for the care of low risk parturient women.

(Cooperative Birth Center Network, 1981)

HISTORY

Birth centers existed in their earliest form not as an alternative to traditional resources of care but as the only available maternity care site and provider in their respective locations for the populations they served. This was true in 1951 when the Certified Nurse-Midwives of Catholic Maternity Institute in Santa Fe, New Mexico began offering maternity care in their birth center as well as in 1972 when the Maternity Unit in Su Clinica Familiar in Raymondville, Texas opened for service.

In the early to mid-1970s an increasing number of families were becoming disenchanted with the traditional physician-hospital mode of maternity care delivery. These families began choosing a do-it-yourself home birth to avoid the traditional course. It was then, in an attempt to address a public health need, that the birth center concept was initiated by the Maternity Center Association of New York. MCA's Childbearing Center began as a demonstration project to evaluate the worth of such an idea that might be also employed to delivery maternity care services in rural or underserved areas. Due to (1) the target population's distrust of hospitals; (2) hospital staff biases; (3) a need to establish the true cost of services; (4) special family requests which might not be met in hospitals with teaching application; and (5) the approval process requirements of the project, the birth center was not designed to be implemented in a hospital setting but instead separated administratively and structurally from a hospital. The development of a home birth service was not a possibility due to the staggering cost of professional staff time for the attendance of a family from the onset of active labor through the early postnatal period and the abundance of crime occurring at all hours of the day within the service area (Lubic, 1976).

PHILOSOPHY OF CARE

Based on the belief that for the majority of childbearing families childbirth is a normal physiologic process and that safe, satisfying, and economic care for childbearing families opting out of the traditional care system can be delivered in a freestanding birth center, the Childbearing Center (CbC) at MCA was established. Essential elements of the CbC model include: (1) the established risk screening criteria for the antenatal, intrapartum, postpartum and neonatal period upon which low risk families are permitted to remain in the Childbearing Center program or be transferred to a back-up physician and/or hospital; (2) quality care delivered by nurse-midwives with expertise in the provision of low risk care with family centered emphasis and a nursing background preparing them to meet the broad spectrum of a family's needs; (3) minimal availability of obstetrical technology, excepting emergency equipment; (4) emphasis on consumer education and participation in care; (5) emphasis on two-way referral pattern with high risk families being referred to high risk facilities and low risk families being referred to the CbC; and (6) an emphasis on quality maternity care for the low risk family offered at as close to cost as possible (Lubic & Ernst, 1978). Since a birth center is not connected structurally or administratively to a hospital, there are no significant cost shifts to accelerate patient charges. As a result, care can often be provided for as low as one-third to one-half the cost of comparable care by a physician and hospital in the community (Lubic, 1979). The FBC charges do not include any recognition of the indirect cost for unused hospital or provider back-up.

FBC services

The realm of services typically provided by birth centers include: pregnancy testing, well woman care, prenatal care, counselling, childbirth education, aspects of self care, intrapartum care, postpartum follow-up, family planning, well baby care, prenatal and postnatal home visiting, and parenting classes. Often families return home within a few hours of their giving birth.

Available technology

Types of high risk technology not generally available in birth centers include antepartum or intrapartum pitocin, spinal, epidural or general anaesthesia, internal fetal monitoring, vacuum extractor, forceps and in some cases, narcotic analgesia. However, emergency equipment for newborn resuscitation or maternal haemorrhage is universally available. If the need for high risk technology arises, transfer of the family to a pre-arranged physician and/or hospital is accomplished. Strict adherence to the use of only a minimum of technology in the FBCs is supported by the recognition of the risk frequently associated with implementation of a particular technology despite its recognized necessity.

Physical location

The physical location of an FBC is clean, warm, homelike and private. It is arranged to best meet the individual family's needs. In addition to homelike birth rooms that accommodate a double bed, family members and emergency equipment, FBCs usually have a kitchen for family use in preparing meals, a living room for visitors as well as separate bathrooms for family and staff. Ideally, the bathroom has a bathtub which can be utilized during labor by clients as desired. There should also be separate work and rest areas for staff use. An emergency area for infant resuscitation, examination room(s), a laboratory area, dirty and clean utility areas, a supply room, office space as well as classroom space are needed. If clinics are held in the FBC, they should be physically separate from the birth rooms in order that adequate privacy be available to the family in labor. All applicable local fire, safety, and health facility codes must be met. Most important, an FBC is not only a physical location but a complete maternity service of which the site is a single aspect.

Professional and institutional support required by FBCs

The service of FBCs is dependent on the total health care system's resources, particularly on the complex medical care system, to receive the FBC's high risk referrals. All FBCs depend on a range of individual facilities and providers in the surrounding community (see Fig. 2.1).

Four states (Oregon, Washington, Pennsylvania and Kansas), as well as the Cooperative Birth Center Network, developed regulations for the licensure of birth centers. Based on these efforts, the American Public Health Association in November 1982 adopted a set of regulations to propose for use nationwide. The purpose of these regulations is to assure the delivery of the highest quality of personalized maternity care for exclusively low risk families at FBCs. They should also ensure appropriately prepared staff work within FBCs with adequate hospital and physician back-up.

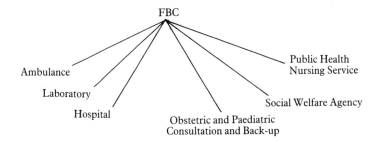

Fig. 2.1

Licensure will also require that the above defined community services are available to FBC patients as needed if not provided by the FBC staff themselves.

SUPPORTIVE CONTEXT FOR GROWTH OF FBCs

The literature

Several areas of research have strongly supported the growth and development of freestanding birth centers. The literature concerns: (1) risk associated with childbearing and the related development of obstetrical risk screening criteria; (2) consumer expectations of the childbirth experience; and (3) the progress of technological development in obstetrics.

Risk associated with childbearing

Several research studies preceded the developments of risk assessment measures for the ascertainment of various antepartum, intrapartum and postpartum maternal and infant conditions associated with subsequent perinatal morbidity or loss. These studies identified single variables that repeatedly were found to be associated with high fetal and perinatal morbidity or mortality. Only in studies beginning after 1960 were combinations of variables considered in these associations.

Lilienfeld & Parkhurst (1951) retrospectively reviewed the birth certificates of 561 children with cerebral palsy born between 1940 and 1947 in New York State who survived the first month of life. The authors found a significant relationship between certain obstetric conditions and cerebral palsy. These conditions included: prematurity, multiple birth, a history of previous stillbirth or infant loss, toxemia or placental abnormalities.

Wells et al (1958) presented the results of a 15-month prospective pilot study which compared medical-obstetric and demographic data of every fetal and neonatal death with a normal infant comparison group at three North Carolina hospitals. The results of the study were that maternal socioeconomic status, age, birth interval, and the length of gestation were all significantly different between the subjects and controls for perinatal death with variants controlled. Of interest was that prenatal care, maternal nutrition, height and parity did not have a significant impact on perinatal or fetal mortality.

In *Perinatal Mortality: The First Report of the British Perinatal Mortality Survey*, Butler & Bonham (1963) described the results of a cross-sectional study comparing factors associated with normal births and births which produced stillbirths or neonatal deaths. The data collection occurred during a one-week period in 1958 for 17 000 live births and over a three-month period in 1958 for 7000 singleton stillbirths and neonatal deaths. This study found the following significant factors associated with perinatal mortality: parity, lack of prenatal care, prolonged labor, short labors, breech presentation, a history of smoking, prematurity, multiple birth, previous stillbirth or infant death, toxemia and placental abnormalities.

Shapiro & Abramowicz (1969) conducted a prospective study in 1958 of biological and environmental factors related to early fetal loss as well as to morbidity and mortality in early childhood. An attempt was also made to identify factors associated with pregnancy loss and congenital abnormalities. The population studied included 12 000 women who were delivered by physicians in a prepaid health plan in New York City. The infants were followed for two years after birth. Data were extracted from medical records and vital records. Results indicated that 18% of pregnancies which progressed to 12 weeks' gestation resulted in a fetal death, 7%; a neonatal death, 1%; a surviving child with a significant congenital defect diagnosed by the second birthday, 6%; or a low birth weight infant, 4%. An additional 7% of pregnancies resulted in early fetal deaths prior to 12 weeks' gestation. Findings also included that women with previous premature birth or fetal death tended to repeat the same phenomenon after 12 weeks' gestation in a subsequent pregnancy, particularly if the intraconceptual interval was short. History of a gynaecological disorder in this pregnancy and a history of bleeding or staining in a prior pregnancy were both associated with an increased risk of loss after 12 weeks' gestation. Non-infectious gynaecological disorders, urinary tract infections, antepartum bleeding, rubella and rising rhesus titers were all associated with increased loss or disability prior to 12 weeks' gestation.

In 1972, Niswander & Gordon, of the National Institute of Neurological Diseases and Stroke, reported the findings of a prospective collaborative study of 55 908 study mothers and their children conducted from 1959 to 1965 in 15 university-affiliated medical centers across the United States. The purpose of this study was to examine the relationship of different variables in the perinatal environment to each other and to the continuum of reproductive failure. Some results of the study were that a maternal history of smoking, parity, infertility, organic heart disease, diabetes, or the presence of urinary tract infections, vaginal bleeding, incompetent cervix, hydramnios, placental abnormalities, prolonged labor, short labor, and breech presentation were strongly associated with perinatal loss.

Kessner et al in 1973 under the auspices of the Institute of Medicine produced a report based on New York City vital statistics data on 140 000 New York City births which occurred in 1968. In the case of infant deaths, birth and death records were linked. Some of the findings included that when obstetric risk and care received were compared across ethnic groups, infant death rates for infants of foreign born white women ranged from 7.4 per 1000 with adequate care and no risk to 68.1 per 1000 for infants of black native-born women with poor care and social and medical risk. When medical risk was controlled and care was adequate, ethnicity made little difference to outcome. The authors reported that risk, care and outcomes are the same for either the neonatal period only or within the entire first year of life. Postneonatal deaths were minimally affected by prenatal care. Another major finding was that infant mortality rates were more closely associated with infant birth weight than any other characteristic of the mother or infant studied. Infant gestation data were not uniformally available in this study. From the results of this investigation, the authors made recommendations for changes in the delivery of maternal and infant health services for the populations studied.

In 1980, Shapiro et al reported an analysis of data collected on 390 425 single live births which occurred in the U.S.A. in 1974–75 resulting in 5084 infant deaths and 4327 surviving one-year-old children. Data were derived from computer tapes and matched birth and death certificates obtained from health departments. Also, a household survey of infants surviving to one year of age was utilized. Differential sampling was done to obtain large numbers of low birth weight infants who had survived to one year. The survey involved an interview with the mother and observations of the child, which included items from the Bayley and Denver Developmental Screening Inventory. Independent variables in the study were race of child, maternal age, maternal education, maternal history of prior fetal loss and a history of previous Caesarean section. The effect of these variables on birth weight was described. It was noted that gestational age would be examined in future analyses. Patterns of relationships between the independent variables and birth weight were then described as they affected neonatal death, delay or congenital abnormality, postneonatal death and other significant illness. Findings indicated that advanced maternal age and maternal history of prior fetal loss were risk factors for infant loss, congenital abnormalities and developmental delay in surviving infants. Young maternal age, low educational attainment and non-white race were associated with increased postneonatal mortality and morbidity.

Risk criteria developed

It was subsequent to the above studies which identified the factors significantly associated with perinatal morbidity and loss that several authors including Apgar (1953), Prechtl (1967), Goodwin et al (1969), Nesbitt & Aubry (1969), Aubry & Pennington (1973), Hobel et al (1973), Stembera et al (1974), Morrison & Olson (1979), Halliday et al (1980) and Fortney & Whitehorne (1982) developed criteria by which the clinician might identify patients who would be at high risk for reproductive casualty with neonatal implications, low birth weight and perinatal death at a later time. These risk prediction systems are based on the thinking that certain cumulative events might affect perinatal outcome and the outcome of infancy *synergistically*. It is the existence of these criteria that have allowed staff at FBCs to discriminate between who is most likely to experience significant morbidity or mortality in pregnancy, labor or postpartum versus those who might safely receive all their care in the specialized out-of-hospital environment of an FBC.

Selwyn, in a recent National Academy of Sciences publication (1982), reviewed 33 articles discussing 19 risk scoring systems written from 1953 to 1980. She pointed out that the authors of the various risk systems assess clinical and demographic factors in one or all of the following periods: antepartum, intrapartum, postpartum, neonatal and infancy. Certain cut points were set for specific populations which determine whether a patient is at low, medium or high risk for one or more of the following outcomes: neonatal or perinatal mortality, neonatal morbidity, preterm gestation, low Apgar score, and intrapartum or postpartum maternal complications. Obviously, whether the information regarding risk is accurate enough and obtained early enough for accomplishing a reduction in morbidity or mortality of human life is the question. The more time periods assessed with the instruments, the better predictability of the screening method itself influences its predictive capability such as (1) the incidence of occurrence of an outcome in a study population for each level of risk being affected by the characteristics of the population group selected for study, and (2) the weighting of a particular risk factor. Also, the need to generalize findings across a study population may affect the predictive accuracy of the screening device.

Selwyn (1982) recommends that separate weighting and scoring systems be developed at least for each age, ethnic group and social level for primigravidas versus multigravidas; advocates attention to reliability of risk criteria application, particularly if applied only once; and individual risk may be quite different from that of the group upon whose characteristics an instrument is based. Successful prediction of pregnancy and intrapartum conditions of the mother as well as neonatal morbidity is limited according to the present literature. The usefulness of weighting schemes because they are influenced by clinical intervention are difficult to evaluate. The perfection of a uniform risk screening criteria will certainly improve the ability of the researcher to compare low risk care delivery under different conditions or in different locations.

Studies continue to be done to attempt to arrive at the perfect set of risk screening criteria to predict with maximum specificity and sensitivity those factors resulting in perinatal morbidity or mortality. However, the various criteria of the extant sytems do at least permit the separation of women and infants requiring the most sophisticated care from those needing the least sophisticated care.

Consumer expectations of the childbirth experience

In the early 1970s, several conferences were held across the United States to discuss what lay people expected from their childbirth experience and maternity care. Reports from these meetings (Lubic, 1972; Disbrow, 1973) indicated that families wanted more personalized care by a provider who respected their needs and desired their participation in care delivery.

Scaer & Korte (1978) conducted a study in Boulder, Colorado in 1976 to determine the services a new area maternity wing at a local hospital should provide. 645 women who had delivered within one year at this hospital were surveyed. Families responded that in retrospect they did not necessarily prefer a hospital delivery; only 51% (n = 230) of La Leche League families and 62% of Prepared Childbirth families (n = 205) preferred the hospital. Numerous other maternity care options were offered to each group of subjects. Families felt that their most important options were keeping the family together during labor and postpartum and a supportive childbirth environment.

Light et al (1976) reported the results of a 'satisfaction' survey they administered to 291 maternity patients delivering spontaneously in five midwestern hospitals. Only 69% of these subjects stated that they believed their physician understood their feelings despite 88.8% expressing satisfaction with their physician's competence. Less than 75% of the subjects reported satisfaction with any aspect of physician-administered care in labor. Physician explanations regarding procedures and medications were considered adequate by only 62% and 58% respectively. In this study, a group of families emerge who might be described as dissatisfied with the degree of participation they were permitted in their own care.

Women's knowledge and interest in alternative maternity facilities were described by Mather (1980). The author reported the results of a community survey conducted in Salt Lake City, Utah. A random sample of women included 100 women of childbearing age not currently pregnant who intended to become pregnant in the next ten years. 50% of the subjects studied had had a prior birth experience. Subjects were asked to complete a three-part questionnaire on birth options. Results indicated that most subjects lacked awareness of the birthing suite or freestanding birth center concept. Home birth was more familiar. After reading a description of each option, the subjects shared a significantly increased interest in using the two new alternatives. They became less willing to use the traditional medical system after learning about alternatives. Fees for care also had an influence on the subjects' decisions. Obviously, families need to be made aware of what options are available to them. Also, availability of an option alone may increase its use.

In 1981 Fullerton completed an assessment of personal and situational differences in 'control' that distinguish those women who chose out-of-hospital delivery sites for childbirth versus who chose hospital sites. A case comparison of 33 pairs of women who chose in-

and out-of-hospital birth sites (self-selected) were matched by age within three years, parity and marital status. All cases and controls had to be of low obstetrical risk. Two instruments were used between 32 and 37 weeks of pregnancy to measure control in selected subjects: (1) the Attitude Toward Issues of Choice Childbearing Scale; and (2) the 18-item Health Locus of Control (Wallston et al, 1978). The women who chose an out-of-hospital setting versus the in-hospital setting differed in that they had a more positive attitude when making a choice over health related situations rather than deferring to chance, luck or fate. The out-of-hospital group saw themselves as the determinant of their own life events.

Cohen (1981) described the results of a postpartum interview administered to 125 women who had selected tertiary hospital care (34), a hospital birthing room (34) and a freestanding birth center (57). He queried consecutive subjects who were willing respondents as to their reasons for selecting a particular site for their birth. Demographic characteristics of the groups were stated to be similar although not controlled. Four major areas of inquiry were explored: responsibility for self, responsibility for infant, family attitudes and feelings regarding characteristics of 'hospital' environment. Control over the birth process and care of the infant was critical to a majority of non-hospital choosers versus none of the tertiary hospital choosers. A reduction in risk-taking related to birth, pain management and infant care was important to a majority of the hospital choosers versus non-hospital choosers to whom this was not important. A distrust of the medical profession was widespread (45%) in the non-hospital group versus almost non-existent (6%) in the tertiary hospital group. A discomfort with hospital routines was common in the non-hospital (68.4%) versus the tertiary hospital group (14.7%). The hospital birth room group typically responded between the tertiary hospital and non-hospital group except in the area of family attitudes and control of baby where they responded very similarly to the non-hospital group. The entire birthing room and non-hospital groups had Lamaze preparation of childbirth versus conventional prenatal classes taken by the majority of the tertiary hospital group. The birthing room group, like the tertiary hospital group, desired less risk taking related to their responsibility regarding the infant than the non-hospital group. Tests of significance were not done. Cohen concluded that these groups, although seemingly quite different, were similar because they chose what they perceived as safe, responsible and positive for themselves and their offspring. Another conclusion might be that every family has different needs associated with childbearing which cannot be met equally well in a single maternity care setting.

The progress of technological development in obstetrics

Research on the development of obstetric technology is particularly pertinent to the growth and development of FBCs. The vast majority of FBCs originated as a result of health care providers and consumers joining to question the trend toward a less personalized birth experience for families with increased use of obstetric intervention.

Devitt (1977) has outlined the history of the movement from home to the hospital of childbirth in America from the 1930s to the 1960s. In 1935, according to Devitt, 37% of U.S. births occurred in-hospital and the remainder at home. As of 1960, 96% of U.S. births took place in the hospital. This action was strongly supported by obstetricians, public health administrators, insurance companies and women of higher socioeconomic strata. Because of the lack of opposition to this trend, the trend continued. It was not until the 1950s with Ashley Montagu and much later in the late 1960s that the consumer movement began to state their opposition to this trend. Consumers questioned whether indeed hospitals were safer than home and if any decrease in infant and maternal mortality could be attributed to hospitals or to other coincidental factors of the period, such as antibiotics, improved nutrition, or child spacing.

In the *Journal of Tropical Diseases*, Haire (1973), the co-director of the International Childbirth Education Association (a group for consumers and providers associated with childbirth education), wrote a treatise evaluating many common obstetrical practices as well as the routine use of high risk technology for all patients whether they experience complications or not. She provided research substantiating many practices and technological interventions as unnecessary or harmful for childbearing families. Some of the common practices she examined were the separation of mother and infant at birth for an extended period of time — up to 24 hours in some cases — perineal shaving for delivery, lithotomy position for delivery and the use of a central nursery. Technology reviewed included: obstetric anaesthesia and analgesia, electronic fetal monitoring, forceps and other interventions.

Since Haire's review of the literature, numerous additional studies evaluating the same common obstetric practices have appeared. The adequacy of support by obstetric staff for family's participation in their care (Cogan, 1980), use of pubic hair shaving (Romney, 1980), enemas on admission in labor (Romney & Gordon, 1981), the restriction of family members' presence during labor or birth (Sosa et al, 1980), including siblings (Anderson, 1979), the restriction of ambulation in labor (Flynn et al, 1978; Williams et al, 1980), artificial rupture of membranes (Liston & Campbell, 1974; Caldeyro Barcia, 1977; General Accounting Office, 1979), the use of the dorsal position in labor, and lithotomy position for delivery (Huovinen & Teramo, 1979), routine use of episiotomy (Banta & Thacher, 1980) and the separation of parents and their infant for the first hour after birth (Klaus & Kennell, 1976; DeChateau & Wibert 1977) continue to be questioned as to their benefit. Possible iatrogenic effects of some of these practices were raised.

In their book, *Benefits and Hazards of the New Obstetrics* (1977), Chard & Richards reviewed the entire spectrum of obstetric technology's pros and cons, substantiating their conclusions with research evidence. The final chapter in their book is entitled, 'Lessons for the Future', in which they reflect on the relationship of this technology to the cost of providing hospital care, consumer pressure, effective performance of care and prevention of perinatal morbidity and loss. They point out that as workloads fall with the declining birth rate, one option obstetrical professionals have is increased intervention in the care of the remaining few patients. The need for uniform application of such obstetrical technology and intervention demands a more thorough investigation according to these authors.

In 1979, a report was released by the staff of the U.S. General Accounting Office entitled, *A Review of Research Literature and Federal Involvement Relating to Selected Obstetric Practices*. This report summarized an in-depth review of the literature available evaluating the benefits and possible risks associated with five obstetrical interventions:

1. Medications used to relieve labor pain
2. Instrument delivery, including forceps and vacuum extraction
3. Electronic fetal monitoring
4. Induction of labor
5. Caesarean section.

The authors felt that the research results were inconclusive. Often, no long term follow-up studies of the infant were available and methodology of studies done to date made them incomparable and often inadequate. Typically, studies were retrospective with little or no attempt to match critical variables by cohort or case or to randomize the intervention under review. Data utilized to assess the value of a procedure were often collected for a different purpose. Despite inadequate evaluation, however, the procedures frequently became widespread. Some of the procedures have even been found to carry substantial risk when inappropriately applied. Certainly, the findings in this review, as in the earlier studies cited for those families expecting no complications of their pregnancy or birth, the possibility of avoiding unnecessary or possibly harmful intervention, might make the FBC setting appear attractive.

RESEARCH AT FBCs

Introduction

Until recently, research concerning the safety and satisfaction associated with FBC care has been limited, partly due to the inability of researchers to randomly assign families to their care situation. Matched pair comparisons have not been completed since hospitals have not been willing to share their data for purposes of this type of comparison. The data on transfers from FBCs have until recently not been uniformly available within or across sites, often for political reasons. Finally the usefulness of the risk criteria utilized by FBCs in determining who will or will not be transferred needs to be carefully evaluated. First, adequate numbers of cases must be available for study in which similar criteria have been applied.

Data

Although much has been written regarding home birth and in-hospital birth centers, only a small amount of literature is available describing freestanding birth centers. Lubic (1977) wrote about preliminary data from the Maternity Center Association's Childbearing Center. She found that the families seeking care were from a cross section of cultural and religious backgrounds. These families were from all walks of life with the highest percentages being from professional and clerical occupations. Of the group of women delivering in the FBCs, 90% were married, 35% were pregnant for the first time, 55% had a $15 000 annual income or less, 20% were without health insurance, 20% were born outside the U.S. and 76% were non-smokers. The mean age of the group was 28 years with a range 16–37 years, and the mean education was 15 completed years of school with a range of 8–22 years. Of another group of 103 patients, Lubic reported that only 3% said cost was the major factor in seeking FBC care. Most of these families stated that the type of experiene the FBC offered was their most significant reason for choosing this type of care.

Seven articles concerning medical-obstetric characteristics of patients receiving care in freestanding birth centers were located in the published literature as of December 1982. Murdaugh (1976) presented data on 754 patients delivered from July 1, 1972 to June 30, 1976 at Su Clinica Familiar-Raymondville, Texas. She reported that 87% of infants delivered had a one minute Apgar score of seven or above. For these 754 infants, the following list of complications resulted: four cephalohematomas, two scleral hemorrhages, two fractured clavicles and two brachial plexus injuries. The infant mortality within the first 24 hours of life for this group was attributed to severe amnionitis in the mother (1), post-maturity (1), and severe anomalies incompatible with life (2). The puerperal morbidity associated with these cases included the following: postpartum hemorrhage (3), endometritis (14), breast infection (9), and rectal-vaginal fistula (1).

In 1977, Nielsen discussed the results of care provided at her Oregon FBC for 152 families from May 21, 1976 to Spring 1977. She described the following findings: 78 FBC spontaneous deliveries with neonates having an Apgar score of 8–10 at one minute, 13 spontaneous abortions, 3 families advised to transfer to high risk obstetrical care, 15 moved out-of-area, 5 lost to follow-up, 12 transfers to home delivery with lay-midwife or another certified nurse-midwife in the area performing home births, and 26 deliveries in a back-up hospital.

In *Nursing Outlook*, Lubic & Ernst (1978) presented a brief summary of the first 300 births which occurred at the Maternity Center Association's Childbearing Center. According to the authors, one-third of the patients who presented for antepartum care were transferred out of the program or withdrew at some point. No cases of placenta abruptio, cord prolapse or postpartum hemorrhage were reported. In two transferred families who suffered a neonatal loss after hospital managed labor, the prior CbC care apparently could not be faulted. One infant died suddenly at home after discharge and was diagnosed as possibly Sudden Infant Death Syndrome. Of nine intrapartum and postpartum transfers reported, the reasons for transfer included: mild respiratory distress (5), birth weight less than 2500 grams (2), appearance of clinical post-maturity (1), and possibility of sepsis (1). Of the infants delivered, 76% had Apgar scores of nine or ten at one minute and 87% had Apgar scores of ten at five minutes.

A second article appearing in the literature concerning the Maternity Center's Childbearing Center (Faison et al, 1979) discussed information on the first 714 women who registered for prenatal care at the Center. Of these women, 28% (199) were parous and 72% (515) were nonparous. 77 women, or 11%, were ineligible for care subsequent to the first visit according to the Maternity Center Association's risk screening criteria. 177 women were referred or transferred prior to delivery for the following reasons: ruptured membranes with no apparent labor within 12 hours, non-vertex presentation, premature labor prior to 37 weeks of gestation, and post-maturity. 58 women were transferred in labor for these reasons: failure to progress in labor (26), fetal bradycardia (2), hypertension (12), non-vertex presentation on intrapartum admission (1), and inspection and general repair under general anaesthesia by a physician (1). Nine infant transfers included birth weight less than 2500 grams (2), clinical post-maturity (1), mild respiratory distress (5), and question of sepsis (1). The mean birth weight of these patients was between 3000 to 3499 grams. None of the 242 infants had an Apgar between four and six at one minute. Exclusive of these patients who transferred, only one family failed to return for a six-week postpartum check-up; they had moved away from the area. No additional known problems resulted from the transfer of the mothers or infants discussed above aside from the two neonatal losses mentioned earlier in the Lubic & Ernst article (1978).

In a subsequent article, Lubic (1980) described the first 1166 families who came to a first antenatal visit at the Maternity Center Association's Childbearing Center. The demographic and event information described was quite similar in pattern to the previous article although further elaboration was given. Of those women completing an initial visit at the CbC, 4% spontaneously aborted, 9% were ineligible ('risked out') at the first visit, 25% were transferred to their back-up physician, 10% withdrew or moved, 39% delivered and 14% remained in the program as of July 1, 1979. Of the transfers to hospital intrapartum, none were due to placental abruption, cord prolapse or hemorrhage. Among those women who began labor under the care of the CbC staff, only 5% required transfer to a hospital and subsequent Caesarean section. No further deaths or untoward events occurred beyond those described in the earlier articles.

An unpublished study conducted by Halle in 1980 on an out-of-hospital birth center involved a center in which care was partially administered by a physician. This physician, a certified nurse-midwife (CNM) and registered nurse each participated in the direct care of families at the center. Unlike most CNM directed sites, certain obstetric technology was routinely available at the center such as pitocin augmentation. Halle reported the results of her prospective matched pair comparison of this freestanding birth center's outcomes with those of a hospital. Both populations were identically risked utilizing the Hobel risk system (POPRAS). Some attempt was made to control socioeconomic characteristics of both populations including race, age, parity and marital status. The investigator summed the total number of intrapartum, postpartum and neonatal risk factors in both groups and compared these numbers using percent and Chi-square analyses. She reported no significant differences in the total number of intrapartum and neonatal risk factors. There was, however, a significant difference (p < 0.01) in the number of postpartum risk factors identified in the two populations to the hospital's advantage. One limitation of the study was, however, that postnatal observations of study subjects were made for up to twice as long in the birth center as in the hospital. Given the rarity of some obstetrical and neonatal events, another major limitation of this study despite equivalent populations was the small sample (43) in each group.

DeJong et al (1981), following a retrospective case review of the first consecutive 180 FBC patients receiving care at Seattle, Washington FBC presented their findings. A major focus of the review concerned the adherence of the FBC staff to adopted risk screening criteria. Only low risk cases were permitted to receive care at the FBC. The authors found an antepartum referral rate of 14% and an intrapartum referral rate of 16%. They also observed that an additional 17% of the FBC's patients would have been transferred had the risk criteria been adhered to precisely. The validity of the screening criteria was confirmed by the higher rates of low one minute Apgar scores and other complications (i.e. amnionitis) of those not transferred. The authors question the cost savings to FBC clients since the back-up hospital assumes indirect costs of care should their services be needed. Further, the author proposes that medical staff committees in hospitals consider modifying criteria for staff privileges in maternity care units to include certified nurse-midwives.

In 1981, Bennetts completed the first national study of a stratified, systematic sample of 1938 low risk women who began labor between 1972 and 1979 in one of the 11 selected nurse-midwifery-directed freestanding birth centers with physician and hospital back-up in the United States. These women were found to be much like those described previously in small single center studies reported in the literature. The mean age was 25 years. 63% were white, 34% Hispanic, 88% married, 45% had completed at least two years of college, nearly one-third were professionals and over a third were housewives. 95% of patients delivered infants at term, usually without complication. Nearly 60% of the FBC labors were unmedicated. 79% of the infants were breastfed. Transfers versus non-transfers were significantly more educated and often without living children. 15% of the FBC patients required transfer to the hospital after the onset of labor due to a change in their risk status. According to the directors of the various sites, 10% required transfer or referral antepartum or were ineligible for care. Further, a rough comparison between these women who began labor in an FBC and 4790 similarly risked women who began labor in a hospital in the United States in 1972 was made. Age, race and gravidity were controlled. Significantly (p < 0.05), more antenatal visits and better postnatal visits compliance was found in the FBC group. Intrapartum anaesthetic use in the hospital sample significantly exceeded that in the FBC sample. No statistically significant difference were found between numbers of neonatal deaths which occurred in the FBC and hospital populations, although the FBCs had proportionately fewer deaths. Portions of this study have been reported in the literature (Bennetts & Ernst, 1982; Bennetts & Lubic, 1982).

A retrospective cohort study was completed by Feldman in 1982 comparing two groups of low risk women matched on age, parity, marital status, high school education, low risk obstetric status as ascertained by Hobel's Risk Criteria (1973) and private insurance coverage. One group of the women received their intrapartum care in an FBC, one in hospital. More interventions were applied in the hospital population and the evidence of some complications were higher in the hospital group. No significant difference in any outcome was found. These results have caused questions to be raised as to whether the use of specific interventions are appropriate when applied routinely to clients not expected to experience obstetrical complications.

CONCLUSIONS FROM FBC DATA

Researchers seem to conclude that FBCs can offer care at least as safely as hospitals to equally low risk families. FBCs can provide an inexpensive alternative to greater than 70% of pregnant women. Currently, somewhat less than 1% of women take advantage of this personalized alternative nationally. The future of FBCs will depend on consumer interest in FBCs and the health care industry's cooperation despite the declining birth rates and increasing numbers of obstetrical providers.

The FBC concept may gradually be moved within the hospital walls if or when hospitals become willing to discontinue their current price structures and alter their approach to the low risk family. This will require a dramatic change in attitudes of hospital-based physicians and nurses toward family-centered care and toward the application of high risk technology. There would also need to be an increased willingness to allow certified nurse-midwives hospital privileges.

REFERENCES

American Public Health Association 1982 Guidelines for licensing and regulating birth centers. Passed by American Public Health Association Governing Council November 17, 1982
Anderson S V 1979 Siblings at birth: A survey and study. Birth and the Family Journal 6(2): 80–87
Apgar V 1953 A proposal for a new method of evaluation of the newborn infant. Current Research in Anaesthesia and Analgesia 32: 260–267
Aubry R H, Pennington J C 1973 Identification and evaluation of high risk pregnancy: The perinatal concept. In Osofsky H J (ed) High risk pregnancy with emphasis on maternal and fetal well-being. Clinical Obstetrics and Gynecology 16: 3–27
Banta D, Thacher D 1980 Benefits and risks of routine episiotomy: An interpretive review of the english language literature, 1960–1980. Center for Disease Control, Atlanta, Georgia
Bennetts A B 1981 Out-of-hospital childbearing centers in the United States: A descriptive study of the demographic and medical-obstetric characteristics of women beginning labor therein: 1972–1979. PhD dissertation (unpublished). University of Texas School of Public Health, Houston, Texas
Bennetts A B, Ernst E K M 1982 Freestanding birth centers. In: Institute of Medicine, National Academy of Sciences, Research issues in the assessment of birth settings. National Academy Press, Washington, D. C.
Bennetts A B, Lubic R W 1982 The freestanding birth center. Lancet 1: 378–380
Butler N R, Bonham D G 1963 Perinatal mortality: The first report of the 1958 British perinatal mortality survey under the auspices of the National Birthday Trust Fund. E. & S. Livingstone, Edinburgh
Caldeyro-Barcia R 1977 Some consequences of obstetrical interference. Birth and the Family Journal 2: 34
Chard T, Richard M 1977 Benefits and hazards of the new obstetrics. Heinemann Medical, London
Cogan R 1980 Effects of childbirth preparation. Clinical Obstetrics and Gynecology 23(1): 2–14
Cohen R L 1981 Factors influencing maternal choice of childbirth alternatives. Journal of the American Academy of Child Psychiatry 20(1): 1–15

Cooperative Birth Center Network 1981 Draft of recommendations for regulatory
  bodies concerned with the licensure of birth centers. Cbcn News 1(1): 3
DeChateau P, Wibert B 1977 Long term effect on mother-infant behavior of extra
  contact during first hour postpartum. Acta Paediatricia Scandinavica 66: 137–151
DeJong R N, Shy K K, Carr K C 1981 An out-of-hospital birth center using
  university referral. Obstetrics and Gynecology 58(6): 703–707
Devitt N 1977 The transition from home to hospital birth in the United States,
  1930–1960. Birth and the Family Journal 4(2): 47–57
Disbrow M (ed) 1973 Meeting consumer demands for maternity care: Conference for
  nurses and other professionals. Seattle, Washington: University of Washington
Ernst K M 1982 Personal communication
Faison J B, Pisani B J, Douglas R G, Cranch G S, Lubic R W 1979 The childbearing
  center: An alternative birth setting. Obstetrics and Gynecology 54: 527–532
Feldman E 1982 Toward improved family health: A comparison of process and
  outcome of childbirth for low risk women in an in-hospital and out-of-hospital
  setting. Medical student paper (unpublished) submitted to Mount Sinai
  Department of Obstetrics, New York City, New York
Flynn A M, Kelly J, Hollins G, Lynch P F 1978 Ambulation in labour. British
  Medical Journal 2: 591–593
Fortney J A, Whitehorne E W 1982 Develpment of an index of high risk pregnancy.
  American Journal of Obstetrics and Gynecology 143: 501–508
Fullerton J D T 1981 The choice of in- or out-of-hospital birth environment as
  related to selected issues of control. Unpublished doctoral thesis submitted to
  Department of Health Education, Temple University, Philadelphia, Pennsylvania
General Accounting Office (DHEW) 1979 A review of research literature and federal
  involvement relating to selected obstetric practices. U.S. General Accounting
  Office, Washington, D.C.
Goodwin J W, Dunne J T, Thomas B W 1969 Antepartum identification of the fetus
  at risk. Canadian Medical Association Journal 101: 458
Haire D 1973 Cultural warping of childbirth. Journal of Tropical Diseases 19:
  171–179
Halle J N 1980 Elective birth center delivery for low risk pregnancy: Effect on
  perinatal outcome. Unpublished thesis presented to the faculty at California State
  University Department of Nursing at Los Angeles
Halliday H L, Jones P K, Jones S L 1980 Methods of screening obstetric patients to
  prevent reproductive wastage. Obstetrics and Gynecology 55(5): 656–661
Hobel C J, Hyvariner N A, Okada D M, Uh W 1973 Prenatal and intrapartum high
  risk screening: I. Prediction of the high risk neonate. American Journal of
  Obstetrics and Gynecology 117: 1–9
Huovinen K, Teramo K 1979 Effect of maternal position of fetal heart rate during
  extradural anaesthesia. British Journal of Anaesthesia 51(8): 767–773
Kessner D M, Singer J, Kalk C E, Schlesinger E R 1973 Infant death: An analysis by
  maternal risk and health care. Institute of Medicine, National Academy of
  Sciences, Washington D.C.
Klaus M H, Kennell J H 1976 Maternal-infant bonding. C V Mosby, St Louis
Light H K, Solheim J S, Hunter G W 1976 Satisfaction with medical care during
  pregnancy and delivery. American Journal of Obstetrics and Gynecology 125:
  827–831
Lilienfeld A M, Parkhurst E 1951 A study of the association of factors of pregnancy
  and parturition with the development of cerebral palsy. American Journal of
  Hygiene 53: 262–282
Liston W A, Campbell A J 1974 Dangers of oxytocin induced labour to fetuses.
  Lancet 3(5931): 606–607
Lubic R W 1972 What the lay person expects of maternity care: Are we meeting these
  expectations? JOGN Nursing 1: 25–31
Lubic R W 1976 Alternative patterns of nurse-midwifery care: I. The childbearing

center: A demonstration project in out-of-hospital care. Journal of Nurse-Midwifery 21: 24–25

Lubic R W 1977 Comprehensive maternity care as an Ambulatory Source-Maternity Center Association's birth alternative. Journal of the New York State Nurses Association 8: 19–24

Lubic R W 1979 Economic aspects of the childbearing center. An unpublished report of the Maternity Center Association, New York City, New York

Lubic R W 1980 Evaluation of an out-of-hospital maternity center for low risk patients. In: Aiken L (ed) Health policy and nursing practice. McGraw-Hill, New York

Lubic R W, Ernst E K M 1978 The childbearing center. An alternative to convention care. Nursing Outlook 26: 754–760

Mather S 1980 Women's interest in alternative maternity facilities. Journal of Nurse-Midwifery 25(3): 3–10

Morrison I, Olson J 1979 Perinatal mortality and antepartum risk scoring. Obstetrics and Gynecology 53: 362–366

Murdaugh S A 1976 Experiences of a new migrant health clinic. Women and Health I

Nesbitt R E L, Aubry R H 1969 High risk obstetrics II: Value of semi-objective grading system in identifying the vulnerable group. American Journal of Obstetrics and Gynecology 103: 972–983

Nielsen I 1977 Nurse-midwifery in an alternative birth center. Birth and the Family Journal 4: 24–27

Niswander K R, Gordon M 1972 The women and their pregnancies. W. B. Saunders, Philadelphia

Prechtl H F R 1967 Neurological sequelae of prenatal and perinatal complications. British Medical Journal 34: 763

Romney M L 1980 Predelivery shaving: An unjustified assault? Journal of Obstetrics and Gynecology 1: 33–35

Romney M L, Gordon H 1981 Is your enema really necessary? British Medical Journal 282: 1269–1271

Scaer R, Korte D 1978 MOM survey: Maternity options for mothers — what do women want in maternity care? Birth and the Family Journal 5: 20–26

Selwyn B J 1982 Review of obstetrical risk assessment methods. In Institute of Medicine, National Academy of Sciences, Research issues in the assessment of birth settings. National Academy Press, Washington, D.C.

Shapiro S, Abramowicz M 1969 Pregnancy outcome correlates identified through medical record based information. American Journal of Public Health 59: 1629–1650

Shapiro S, McCormick M C, Starfield B H, Krischer J P, Bross D 1980 Relevance of correlates of infant deaths for significant morbidity at one year of age. American Journal of Obstetrics and Gynecology 136(3): 268–373

Sosa R, Kennell J, Klaus M, Robertson S 1980 Effects of a supportive companion on perinatal problems, length of labor, and mother-infant interaction. New England Journal of Medicine 303: 597–600

Stembera Z K, Zezulokova J, Dittrichova J 1974 Identification and quantification of high risk factors affecting fetus and newborn. Proceedings of the 4th European Congress of Perinatal Medicine, Prague, 28–31

Wallston K A, Wallston B S, DeVellis R 1978 Development of the Multidimensional Health Locus of Control (MHLC) Scales. Health Education Monographs 6(2): 160–170

Wells H B, Greenberg B C, Donnelly J F 1958 North Carolina fetal and neonatal death study I — study design and some preliminary results. American Journal of Public Health 48: 1583–1595

Williams R M, Thom M H, Studd J W W 1980 A study of the benefits and acceptability of ambulation in spontaneous labour. British Journal of Obstetrics and Gynaecology 87: 122–126

Management and nursing care in high risk pregnancy

INTRODUCTION

The term 'high risk pregnancy' means that pregnancy involves an above-average risk to the mother, or fetus, or both. Any one factor, or a combination of factors, may give rise to this situation. A high risk pregnancy is one in which the fetus has an above-average chance of death, either before or after birth and/or a greater probability of later disability (Bibeau & Perez, 1980), or is one which creates a health risk to the mother. Careful evaluation of signs and symptoms is needed to establish a diagnosis, complemented, where necessary, by biophysical feedback and electronic monitoring of mother and fetus. But the procedures required to arrive at a diagnosis, including the tests, place an added strain on parents during pregnancy and may complicate the normal course of psychological preparation for parenthood. It is important, however, to remember that healthy reproduction is the norm and that most mothers identified as being at minimum risk in early pregnancy will proceed to normal delivery of a healthy child. It follows that women who have a low-risk assessment in early pregnancy should not be subjected to unnecessary tests and procedures when there is no medical reason for doing so.

Increased ability to identify and monitor the mother and/or fetus at risk has resulted in decreasing perinatal death rates and decreased morbidity in the last decade. As new facilities have been provided and new tests and equipment introduced, nurses have had to be trained to monitor the mother and fetus in new and innovative ways. The high technology involved in these new monitoring devices has, at the same time, created the risk that parents will view maternity care as increasingly depersonalized and lacking in human values. For the mothers the development of high risk centres often means separation from family and friends, as they have to leave their own environment to undergo surveillance in a large urban centre. Additional psychosocial stresses are thus added to those experienced during normal pregnancy. The nurse's role in guidance, support and education for the at-risk family may be critical to the successful outcome of the pregnancy.

Maternal history

Critical factors in a pregnancy history include the general physical and demographic characteristics of the parents, any co-existent maternal, medical or surgical disorders, past reproductive performance and any complications of the current pregnancy.

A pregnancy history commences with a family history, with particular emphasis placed on any history of problems in pregnancy, labour and delivery, as these can be predictive of a potential for problems during the current pregnancy. The medical history identifies the mother's potential for any chronic disease likely to affect the pregnancy. A family history of previous children with problems that may be genetic or chromosomal in origin is important. A social history should include age, marital status, income, education, religion and ethnic affiliation.

CLINICAL ASSESSMENT AND EVALUATION

Clinical assessment refers to information obtained primarily through physical examination, observation, palpation, percussion, auscultation and measurement. The purpose of this examination is to confirm healthy bodily function and to detect disease and disorder. While it may be performed by midwives and nurses having skill in performing physical examinations, usually the initial physical examination is performed by a physician. Knowledge of normal biology, psychology and sociology of pregnancy and historical data on the mother's family, together with the findings from the physical assessment, provide the foundation for nursing care of the pregnant family.

Physical examination of all systems will be completed at the initial visit. The nurse should endeavour to decrease the patient's embarrassment and fear by discussing the procedures to be used and explaining their purpose, and should promote relaxation by ensuring privacy and creating a trusting climate.

If there is a history of previous stillbirths or a congenital anomaly, it is probable that parents will receive genetic counselling. An amniocentesis may be advised so that chromosomal studies may be undertaken to determine whether or not the fetus is normal. Ultrasound scanning may also be recommended as some types of anomaly may be detected early by this technique.

Ultrasound has been used in first trimester to establish that a pregnancy exists, to diagnose hydatidiform moles; to demonstrate neural tube defects and to identify multiple pregnancy (Garrett & Robinson, 1970). In the very early period of pregnancy it is possible that the sound waves could disturb cell alignment in newly forming tissues (Bolsen, 1982). Findings in rats have shown fetal aberrations when ultrasound is used during early development (Health and Welfare, Canada, 1982). This suggests the need for caution in using ultrasound, although it is recognized that one cannot extrapolate findings directly from rat to human embryos. However, these findings suggest that ultrasound should be limited to those mothers where a diagnosis is needed to determine optimal management. The lessons learned from indiscriminate use of diagnostic X-rays must be remembered when using any new technique.

Abnormal clinical findings

On the first visit it is important to note accurately the baselines for all vital signs. One critical dimension during abdominal examination is to establish the relationship of uterine growth to the last known menstrual period. In some studies incompatibility between menstrual history and uterine growth has been found to be a good predictor of potential perinatal problems (Rayburn, 1982). If the uterus is small for dates in the first trimester it may be that the mother has recalled incorrectly the dates of her last normal period or a fetal anomaly may be developing. If the uterus is large for dates there may be a possibility of hydatidiform mole or multiple pregnancy. Consistency of the uterine size with the last normal menstrual period is the best non-invasive way of measuring fetal growth (Mann et al, 1974; Behrman, 1977). If the mother is seen later in her pregnancy and is found to have a uterus smaller than anticipated based on her medical history, careful serial clinical examinations of uterine height will be needed. Such examinations have been shown as diagnostic for 30–50% of growth-retarded fetuses (Battaglia, 1970; Cook, 1977; Tejani & Mann, 1977). Serial measurement of girth, while used less frequently, may also be used to identify potential problems.

Intrauterine growth retardation is caused by two basic mechanisms. The first is a primary reduction in fetal growth due to lack of nutrients from the mother transplacentally. This may be associated with maternal malnutrition or placental malfunction. The second mechanism is a secondary reduction in fetal growth following a period of normal growth and is commonly related to genetic disorders or infections. Whatever the cause, early detection is critical as the potential for intrauterine asphyxia and death is high if the unsatisfactory status of the fetus remains undetected for too long.

Measurement

Maternal and fetal vital signs should be measured at each prenatal visit. Normally the fetal heart cannot be heard by auscultation before the 24th week but can be identified by the 10th week by using the Doptone or other electronic monitor.

A maternal blood pressure of +30/15 mmHg over a recorded normotensive base line or a mean arterial pressure of greater than 90 mm in the second trimester or greater than 100 mmHg in the third trimester are significant. The nurse should screen the patient further for signs of proteinuria or edema. The 'roll over' test may be used to predict the development of gestational hypertension. In the 'roll over' test an initial blood pressure reading is taken with the woman lying on her left side, then she rolls on to her back and a second measurement is taken when the blood pressure is stable. A diastolic reading that is more than 20 mmHg higher in the second position, compared to the first, is a warning signal and has been found to be a reasonably accurate predictor of preeclampsia (Verma et al, 1980). It can be performed on all mothers between 28–34 weeks gestation and should be performed on those at risk for uterine growth failure, that is, mothers with a history of essential hypertension, cardiac or chronic renal disease, drug or alcohol abuse, excessive smoking or viral infections.

Maternal weight gain

For many years a recommendation was made that weight gain in pregnancy should be limited to 20–24 pounds, with a gain of no more than a pound a week in the last trimester. More recent experience has cast doubt on the wisdom of this advice. A mother who starts pregnancy in a malnourished state may well starve the developing fetus. Today greater emphasis is placed on the manner in which weight is gained. A weight curve which accelerates in the last trimester, but which shows no peaks or valleys, is considered to demonstrate normal fetal growth (Tejani et al, 1976). In the third trimester a lack of weight gain over a two week period in the absence of maternal illness could well be indicative of problems in the fetal-placental unit and would suggest a failure in fetal growth. Such a plateau would alert the midwife or physician to the need to consider ultrasound scanning to determine fetal growth.

BIOCHEMICAL DIAGNOSIS AND EVALUATION

At initial screening, blood type and Rh factor should be determined, as well as hematocrit and haemoglobin levels. Serology screening for syphilis is usually routine. In some countries routine screening for rubella antibody levels is done. While immunization is contra-indicated in pregnancy, a baseline titre is useful if a rubella contact occurs in early pregnancy. Preferably all women should be screened prior to pregnancy and if the titre is less than 1:10, they should be immunized. However, pregnancy should be prevented for a minimal period of two months following such immunization.

If urinary glycosuria is present, either a fasting or postprandial blood sugar should be obtained and if this is abnormal a glucose tolerance test may be indicated before gestational diabetes can be ruled out. Glycosuria is present in about 30% of pregnancies and may be related to a decreased renal threshold or increased resistance to insulin. Because of the risk of maternal diabetes to the developing infant, gestational diabetes should be ruled out before these other causes are assumed.

Urine is tested for protein and sugar using a dipstick or a clean catch specimen. A laboratory specimen should be examined for bacteria and casts if protein is present. The presence of more than 1 g protein/24 hour period in urine indicates renal disorder of some type.

PSYCHOSOCIAL ASSESSMENT

Physiological and psychosocial assessment do not occur in isolation. Psychosocial assessment may provide additional insight into potential physiological problems.

It is critical to determine whether or not the mother wants the baby and the degree of anxiety she has in relation to any potential problem and her understanding of the obstetrician's explanation of that problem. Acceptance of an abnormal fetus may be influenced by such factors as age, cultural orientation, religious beliefs and socioeconomic status. To be supportive the nurse must determine the importance of these factors to each client. No judgment regarding a client's behavior can ever be made until assumptions are verified with the pregnant mother and, if appropriate, her husband (or partner). There is also a need to assess the mother's support system, particularly the husband's response to a problem pregnancy. The initial psychosocial assessment by the nurse may provide guidelines for later nursing management.

Following the history and physical examination, all information should be studied for identification of potential risk factors. A prediction of the incidence of problems and the potential outcome of the risk threat should be made. In this way early diagnosis of the potential jeopardy for mother-fetus and neonate will be established and an evaluation of the degree of risk to the family can be made.

IDENTIFICATION OF RISK FACTORS

Certain factors are generally accepted as placing the pregnant woman and her fetus at risk, although institutions may weight the various factors differently. Pre-existing medical diseases, such as diabetes, chronic hypertension, or renal disease may be exacerbated by pregnancy and can create a risk to the fetus. Previous obstetrical factors (such as high multiparity; previous complicated delivery; previous stillbirth; history of prematurity or an abnormal fetus) that may have implications for the current pregnancy, are assessed. Certain infectious diseases that can affect the fetus, such as syphilis, genital herpes, rubella nd toxoplasmosis, increase the risk of fetal anomaly. Nutritional factors include obesity or low pregnancy weight as well as low weight gain during pregnancy. Use of certain drugs, whether prescribed, purchased over the counter, or obtained illegally, may be harmful to the fetus. In the prescribed group steroids, anticoagulants, anticonvulsants, diuretics and some antibiotics such as tetracycline, must all be viewed with suspicion. Excess aspirin has been implicated in thrombocytopenia in the newborn while marijuana, heroin and PCP are all known to affect newborn behavior.

Some screening instruments are beginning to give more weight to psychosocial risks. Age has long been recognized as a factor in successful pregnancy outcome, with those younger than 19 or more than 35 being considered at greater risk than the average population. We are beginning to recognize the importance of other factors, such as low income (which may be linked to nutrition), living conditions, educational level, support systems, and previous psychiatric disturbance. Reproductive risk is also more likely in women whose mothers have a history of complications in pregnancy and this information should be sought when obtaining an initial history.

As pregnancy progresses, antepartum bleeding, in either the first trimester or later, raises the risk factor as does hypertension associated with the pregnancy. Multiple pregnancy, or malpresentation of the fetus are also related obstetrical risks.

OCCUPATIONAL HAZARDS

With mothers continuing to work during pregnancy, occupational hazards must be considered in relation to pregnancy. For women working in factories, noise may be a potential hazard. Hartoon & Treuting (1981) report on stress reactions to loud noises and point out that data on the effects of noise on pregnancy are hard to obtain because of the ethical dilemmas inherent in exposing mothers to loud noises. In recent experiments with animals two factors have been identified that related to pregnancy. The first is that prolonged loud noise decreased fertility by stimulating the secretion of gonadotrophins. The second finding, confirmed by several researchers, is that prolonged noise results in more stillbirths, a greater incidence of prematurity and an increase in congenital malformations (Ishii & Yokoburi, 1960; Siegel & Smookler, 1973). When noise was coupled with an additional stress (in this instance, trypan blue), the incidence of anomalies increased. Thus, while these findings are not directly applicable to humans, observation of women who work in noisy environments is critical in order to determine if noise has an adverse effect on human development.

Another potential problem area is the use of videoscreens and their impact on pregnancy. With increasing use of word processing machines by secretaries and the use of visual terminals by computer operators, nurses must be alert to the potential hazards these can pose to the pregnant worker. Sources of radiation within the home must also be observed with care. As a greater array of appliances (such as microwave ovens), using more sophisticated technology, becomes available to the homemaker, so more hazards are introduced into the home environment.

In the work place, exposure to toxic substances, such as chemicals, must continue to be of concern. Community and occupational health nurses must be aware of potential fetal teratogens and ensure that female workers are aware of the risks that they take should pregnancy occur.

SOCIAL POISONS

The two major social poisons are smoking and alcohol. There is evidence that heavy smoking causes growth retardation in utero. Babies born to women who smoke have found to be 200 g lighter on average than babies born to non-smokers. While this reduction in birthweight may not by itself be significant, the incidence of preterm births, fetal anomalies and stillbirths is also higher in mothers who are heavy smokers (Simpson, 1957; Miller & Hassaneim, 1978). The decrease in fetal growth is probably brought about by decreased uterine blood flow and decreased placental amino acid uptake caused by high maternal nicotine levels. One handicap is that research has not shown what level of cigarette smoking causes problems — the term 'heavy smoker' remains undefined.

A similar problem exists in relation to alcohol intake. The term 'fetal alcohol syndrome' has been coined to identify babies born to alcoholic mothers with a range of specific mental and physical abnormalities. It is known that alcohol ingested by the mother reaches the fetus in similar concentrations to that found in maternal serum levels. What is not known is whether some developing fetuses are more sensitive to alcohol than others. We cannot, therefore, adequately advise mothers on the advisability of even one social drink. Generally, newborns with fetal alcohol syndrome have a low IQ, which does not improve with age, and remain physically behind children of the same age level. As the effects of alcohol have probably harmed the fetus early in the developmental period, pre-pregnancy education is needed if fetal damage is to be prevented.

The importance of accurate history taking to identify risk factors as early in pregnancy as possible, cannot be overemphasized. Close monitoring of the mother and fetus can, in many instances, prevent a minimal risk problem from becoming more severe.

RISK SCORING

Assessment of risk is an ongoing process that begins at the initial pregnancy visit and in many settings is a formal part of the pregnancy work-up. A risk screening protocol is completed at designated times during the pregnancy. While the actual scoring system differs greatly from one settng to the next, the aim of all systems is to identify whether the mother and fetus are at high, moderate or low risk as pregnancy progresses and labour approaches. The terms are used to describe the complexity and number of variables affecting or contributing to reproductive outcome. Many scoring tools have been developed to help identify those mothers whose fetus falls within the 'at risk' group. All are useful, but what needs to be considered is that at any time on the reproductive risk continuum the mother, fetus, neonate or family may be at different levels of risk. Thus assessment is an ongoing process from the first prenatal visit and throughout labour and delivery. The measure of success of monitoring is identified by evaluating the status of the newborn and the parents in the postnatal period.

Reassessment near to term, or at the onset of labour, is important so that additional risk factors, which have developed during pregnancy, may be incorporated in the assessment. Such factors as a discrepancy between dates and uterine growth, vaginal spotting, hypertension of pregnancy or emotional trauma may all increase the maternal-fetal risk factors. Examples of screening protocols can be found in many obstetrical nursing and midwifery textbooks.

MONITORING THE MATERNAL-FETAL UNIT

As can be seen, management of a high risk pregnancy, once diagnosed, becomes a matter of monitoring both mother and developing fetus. It must be remembered that in a pregnancy considered to be at risk the threat to mother or fetus may not be equal and that the degree of risk may alter throughout the course of the pregnancy. Thus careful monitoring is required to ensure that normal fetal growth is occurring. Two ways of measuring fetal well-being and growth are through placental estriol secretion and the use of ultrasonography.

ASSESSMENT OF FETAL WELL-BEING

Estriol assessment

Fetal androgen precursors are converted to estriol by the placenta, are further conjugated in the maternal liver and are excreted through the maternal kidneys. Estriol synthesis increases with pregnancy and shows a marked acceleration in production in the third trimester. The excretion of estriol has been found to correlate well with fetal size (Avery, 1975). A diminished estriol secretion is a result of two factors: (1) diminished production of fetal androgen precursors and (2) diminished placental conversion. It has been shown that chronically low estriols are connected to intrauterine growth retardation. In mothers considered to have an at-risk pregnancy, 24 hour urinary estriols are recommended at 32–33 weeks of pregnancy and 35–37 weeks of pregnancy to identify potential growth retardation. While normal estriol levels do not rule out growth retardation it is unlikely that the fetus is severely compromised. Falling estriol levels are a potentially ominous sign of fetal distress and usually indicate a need for immediate further investigation such as a non-stress test.

Some drugs, such as ampicillin, corticosteroids, cascara and methenamine mandelate can produce false positives. If the mother has a renal problem, blood serum assays may need to be used instead of urinary estriols.

Collecting urine for estriols is a challenge for most women, as a 24 hour specimen is needed. The nurse needs to review the reasons for the study and to relay any 'tips' she has learned from other women. It is possible to obtain and provide containers that fit under the toilet seat at home. Another tip which eases the chore of collection is to suggest making or obtaining a cover for a quart mayonnaise jar when serial estriols must be collected. This allows the mother to visit friends and continue to collect specimens without embarrassment. A sense of trust between the mother and nurse will also encourage accuracy in reporting if any urine is lost in the 24 hour period (Cranley, 1979).

Ultrasound

As previously mentioned, ultrasound can be used early in pregnancy to determine the presence or absence of specific fetal anomalies. It may also be used to assess fetal growth. Serial fetal cephalometry has important applications in evaluating fetal growth potential. It is frequently used when clinical evidence, such as failure in uterine growth rate, or lack of weight gain, indicates a potential problem. A diagnosis of growth retardation can be based on serial estimates but head growth will usually not start to lag until 34–36 weeks gestation because of brain sparing effects. Some estimates for false negatives are as high as 21% when the biparietal diameter is the only criterion used (Butnarescu et al, 1980). The relationship of head circumference to chest circumference may prove to be of value in identifying the growth retarded fetus. Intrauterine death may also be diagnosed using ultrasound. Because of the possibility of an unfavourable outcome of an ultrasound test, the presence of a nurse, known to the mother, can be of great value in helping her accept the diagnosis and in expressing her initial grief feelings. In one hospital in London a nurse performs the ultrasound scan so she can provide counselling and support at the time of diagnosis.

For some mothers visualisation of the biparietal diameter may be a key factor in helping them to acknowledge that the fetus is real and developing. This is an area where the nurse can help by using test results to encourage women at high risk to identify with the fetus.

BIOPHYSICAL PROFILE SCORING OF THE FETUS

Initial methods for estimating fetal health were based on a single variable. Today a composite measure of observations is used to develop a biophysical profile of the fetus (Manning et al, 1982).

Monitoring of fetal movement

In a 1981 study of 203 women with high risk pregnancy it was reported that the monitoring of fetal activity by the mother provided a 'reliable alternative' to heart rate testing (Rayburn, 1982). When both maternal observation of fetal movement and the stress test indicated danger to the fetus, only one in ten pregnancies had a favourable outcome. If there is some doubt about the degree of fetal movement, mothers can be provided with a chart and asked to record fetal movement when they feel it occurring over a 24 hour period (Hoffmaster, 1978; Coleman, 1981). This is relatively simple for the mother to do, and seems to be a useful preliminary diagnostic tool. If the mother thinks she has decreased movement, or if the recording seems to support this, then a non-stress test is generally advised.

Non-stress test

In a non-stress test an external fetal monitor is applied to the woman's abdomen. The normal test period extends over 20 minutes; if no fetal movement is observed in this period then fundal pressure is applied. No attempt is made to identify other stimuli such as loud noises or bright lights, which have been reported as being potential fetal stimulants. A reactive test is one in which the fetal heart accelerates in response to movement and this is considered a positive sign. A non-reactive test frequently leads to a stress test with induced uterine contractions. For a test to be considered reactive two or more adequate heart rate accelerations should be apparent in the 20–40 minute test period. The amplitude of the reaction should be

15 beats per minute, lasting a minimum of 15 seconds (Rayburn et al, 1982). Primary indications for testing include reports of decreased fetal movement, post maturity, hypertension, maternal diabetes and suspected fetal growth retardation. In Rayburn's (1982) study two-thirds of all non-reactive tests later became reactive or were followed by a reactive oxytocin challenge test. The lack of reaction appeared to be correlated to drugs, cigarette smoking or maternal food intake. It could also be related to a fetal rest period at the time of the study. Rayburn and his colleagues suggest that if no fetal movement is observed during the test period it should be repeated the same day.

The non-stress test is the single method most frequently used and while having a low false negative rate (8 per 1000) it carries both a high false positive rate (75%) and a high incidence of fetal loss with a non-reactive test (perinatal mortality 18 per 1000) (Evertson et al, 1979; Schiffrin, 1982). The test is advantageous in that it is simple to perform, causes no additional stress to the fetus and can be run by a nurse experienced in fetal monitoring.

When the test was first used fetal movement was not recorded on the test strip. Now, all movement, whether felt by the nurse or noted by the mother, is being recorded. This may increase the accuracy of the results. Plastic strips are also being produced that can be placed over the tracing to identify baseline variability, decelerations and beat-to-beat variability. This will decrease error in reading and interpreting the strips.

Stress test or oxytocin challenge test

The purpose of the oxytocin challenge test is to measure fetal reaction in relation to contractions. Evidence of fetal well-being is present when there is no sign of deceleration with the contraction. The contractions are induced by the administration of oxytocin, commonly 2 units of syntocinon in 1000 cc 5% dextrose and water is used. The protocol for administering the syntocinon differs from unit to unit but the principle is to administer just enough oxytocin to stimulate the uterus to contract. If an overdose is given, true labour could be induced and stimulation of premature labour is always a risk with this procedure.

The oxytocin challenge test assesses the response of the fetal heart rate to induced contractions. There is some difficulty in the accuracy with which the test results are interpreted. In one study (Peck, 1980), only 50% agreement was reached as to whether or not fetal

reaction was observed. There is indication of a relatively high incidence of false positives to the oxytocin challenge test. Unlike the
non-stress test, a positive reaction indicates a compromised fetus;
here the emphasis is on the reaction of the fetal heart to a contraction
and a positive test is indicated if decelerations occur. Frequently
there is a lack of correlation between a positive oxytocin challenge
test and placental estriol levels (Weingold et al, 1975).

A negative oxytocin challenge test is generally a reliable indicator
of fetal well-being. Some researchers feel that the oxytocin challenge
test is more sensitive to fetal compromise than urinary estriols.
However, others report a high false negative rate and fetal death has
been reported during a negative test. The false positive rate has been
reported in the range of 50% to greater than 90% (Gauthier et al,
1979).

Because of the high false-positive rate, retesting is frequently
needed. The procedure is not without hazard, in that premature
labour may occur, following the oxytocin-induced contractions.
Manning et al (1982) suggest that when non-stress testing, contraction stress testing and fetal breathing movements are all assessed,
most of the false-positive stress tests are eliminated.

Fetal breathing

Fetal breathing movements are observed during an ultrasound scan.
For a normal score at least 1 breathing episode of 30 seconds'
duration over a 30 minute observation of the fetus must be observed.
An abnormal score results if no episode of breathing is observed in a
30 minute time period.

Amniotic fluid volume

Qualitative measurement of amniotic fluid during ultrasound has
also been used to assess fetal well-being. At least one pocket of
amniotic fluid that measures at least one cm in two perpendicular
planes is required for a normal score. Anything less than this results
in an abnormal score being assigned.

Manning et al report that the false negative rate for a compromised
fetus, using the complete biophysical profile, is less than one per
1000 and when perinatal mortality is corrected for lethal congenital
anomalies, the perinatal mortality has been reduced to 3.5 per 1000
births (Manning et al, 1982). In this Manitoba study the combined
use of real-time B mode ultrasound and Doppler ultrasound assess-

ment did reduce perinatal mortality and also resulted in improved detection of fetal anomaly. An incidental finding was the detection of fetus at risk for acute asphyxia. This group has virtually abandoned the use of urinary estriols and rarely use oxytocin challenge tests. There has also been a 60% reduction in inpatient admission for high-risk pregnancies. They also report that the assurance of fetal well-being provided by the profile has decreased premature intervention with the subsequent risks of failed induction and increased Caesarean section. There are limitations with the method. The exact relationship of duration and degree of insult in relation to fetal symptoms is unknown. The interval between testing that should be utilized is not yet determined. There have been instances when a fetus demonstrated an initial abnormal score, recovered and a healthy newborn was delivered at term. Notwithstanding these problems, the scoring system has potential as a prognostic instrument. The scoring system is outlined in the article written by Manning et al (1982). It would appear that the use of the biophysical profile will be helpful as a diagnostic tool in identifying those pregnancies where intervention to terminate the pregnancy is essential to fetal or newborn survival.

Determination of fetal maturity by the use of biochemical tests

If the fetus appears to be in difficulty in utero, a decision must be made regarding immediate delivery. Generally additional data on fetal maturity are secured to assess the likelihood of respiratory problems arising due to immaturity, particularly of the fetal lungs. The most common test for immaturity is the ratio of lecithin to sphingomyelin in the amniotic fluid.

Lecithin-sphingdomyelin ratio

Pulmonary lung maturity is related to both alveolar and capillary growth and the production of surface active material (surfactant) in the lungs. A deficiency of surfactant has been found in the lungs of newborn dying of hyaline membrane disease (Avery & Mead, 1959).

The measurement of fetal lung maturity is based on the ratio of lecithin to sphingomyelin. An L/S ratio of 2/1 is generally taken as representing fetal lung maturity. Different procedures in laboratories may create variations and as a consequence some institutions will set different ratios (Strassner & Nochimson, 1982). The L/S ratio is generally regarded as the standard test for fetal lung maturity but respiratory distress syndrome may still occur in about 3% of cases evaluated as mature. Caution must be used in interpreting results when the mother is diabetic as elevated L/S ratios are seen while fetal lung immaturity persists.

The Shake test is a rapid test used to determine the presence of surfactant. The test is based on the ability of pulmonary surfactant in amniotic fluid to form a stable foam in the presence of ethanol. A positive (mature) result at a 1:2 dilution of amniotic fluid is a good predictor of absence of respiratory distress syndrome. A high false negative rate is a common occurrence. Contamination of the fluid by blood or meconium can also result in false positives (Strassner & Nochimson, 1982). Any test which is invasive into the uterus carries risks. The first is puncture of the placenta, the second risk is stimulation of the uterus leading to premature labour. It is critical that ultrasound be used to localise the placenta prior to amniocentesis. If the mother has an O-negative blood group, bleeding prior to delivery can cause Rh sensitization and the need for iso-immune gamma globulin should be considered. This has sometimes been overlooked, leading to elevated titres in subsequent pregnancies.

Diagnosis of fetal age by ultrasound

The diagnosis of fetal age has been another major use of ultrasound. Two modes of determination have been used: the crown-rump length of the fetus, which has been used for the sixth to the fourteenth week, and the biparietal diameter before 30–32 weeks gestation. One of the difficulties in using the biparietal diameter is that differences exist in ultrasonic modes used to measure this diameter which has created problems with interpretation (Hughey, 1980). Another difficulty has been in the production and use of charts relating gestational age and biparietal diameter. Specific charts must be used for specific types of ultrasound application. When comparable methods are used and standardized findings applied, no significant differences in measurement of biparietal diameter across different populations by different investigators were demonstrated (Hughey, 1980). Furthermore, gestational age is distributed around a given biparietal diameter in a normal curve so a single estimate of normal growth in relation to gestational age through measurement of the biparietal diameter will tend to be inaccurate if used in the third trimester of pregnancy. The normal variation of a third trimester biparietal diameter appears to be ±3 weeks, thus ultrasound should never be used alone to diagnose gestational age.

Ultrasound has also been used to estimate fetal weight, but indications are that it is no more accurate than clinical estimates obtained through abdominal palpation. Medical management in the prenatal period ends with safe delivery. Based on clinical assessment the mother may progress to normal labour, be induced or be delivered by Caesarean section. The outcome measurement of nursing management may well be the psychological status of the family at the end of the pregnancy.

THE EFFECT OF AN AT RISK PREGNANCY ON THE MOTHER'S SELF-ESTEEM

Over the last few years much has been written on maternal-fetal attachment behaviours in normal pregnancy (Caplan, 1957; Rubin, 1961, 1957; Colman, 1969; Colman & Colman, 1973). This attachment has been described as the psychological work of pregnancy and its completion is believed to be related to a woman's self-esteem. Maternal fetal behaviours in normal pregnancy have been grouped into five categories: role taking; giving of oneself to the fetus; differentiating self from fetus; attributing characteristics to the fetus; and interacting with the fetus (Cranley, 1981). If prenatal attachment behaviour does not occur there is some evidence to show that maternal-fetal attachment postnatally may be delayed. Maternal-fetal behaviours develop as a sequence of events over time (Snyder, 1979). The development takes the form of a trajectory and provides the basis on which maternal expectations of the fetus and newborn are defined and from which maternal behaviour is derived.

In an 'at risk' pregnancy a mother's expected trajectory may alter in relation to the characteristics of her physiological pregnancy, her self-image, her family support system and the interaction she has with the social system that surrounds her. Identification of the trajectory of the at risk mother and comparison with the normal pattern described by Snyder (1979) allows the nurse to diagnose whether or not there is a need for intervention.

An emotional affiliation with the fetus usually indicates that the parents have developed positive hopes and dreams for the unborn child and have a desire for a visual image of the baby (Penticuff, 1982). If the mother gains weight satisfactorily and the pregnancy becomes apparent to others, the mother develops a positive self-image. When a couple have a fetus that is in jeopardy they may be confronted with negative signs, such as failure to gain weight or other signs of intrauterine growth retardation, that threaten the women's self-image. Threats to a woman's sense of self-adequacy seem to affect the maternal-fetal attachment behaviour.

In all pregnancies certain family tasks, such as establishing a home and providing financial support for the family unit, continue. The amount of energy needed by the family for such tasks will determine the amount of energy left to the mother to devote to her relationship with her unborn child (Bodnar, 1982). The presence of older children in the home will also influence the time and energy the mother has left to concentrate on the developing fetus.

Usually when the pregnancy starts to show and the fetus moves, the mother finally recognizes that she is going to have a baby. However, if a woman has lost a previous child, she may ignore the signs and deny the existence of this baby as a protection against being hurt again. If the previous loss was attributable to prematurity a behaviour shift toward developing a relationship with the fetus may occur once the pregnancy has passed the critical point where the previous loss occurred (Bodnar, 1982). However, this is not always the case and observation for maladjustment in maternal-fetal bonding is critical.

When mothers are hospitalized, boredom, powerlessness in the hospital situation and loss of privacy all contribute to stress. Powerlessness, in particular, should be of major concern to nurses. It can be defined as the expectation held by the individual that his own behaviour cannot determine the outcome he seeks (Seeman, 1959).

In order to overcome a feeling of powerlessness, trust must be built up between the perinatal team (physicians and nurses) and the parents. Careful explanation of all recommended tests and procedures with an explanation of their benefits and risks is critical. There must be a commitment to allowing parents to make decisions and for staff to live with the decisions if they are based on presented facts. If a partnership is established between parents and team, feelings of helplessness, with subsequent risk of alienation and hostility, will be decreased (Cranley, 1979).

The mother frequently does not have private time for thinking, dreaming or fantasizing about the baby or her mothering role in the hospital setting. This again militates against the completion of normal maternal-fetal relationship tasks. It is critical that nurses are sensitive to the mother's needs at this time. Provision of information about the pregnancy, the purpose of the tests and the outcomes is essential. Opportunities that promote fetal attachment, such as observing fetal parts during ultrasonography, must be used by nurses. The need to ensure privacy when the husband visits is also critical for promotion of the family support system. When separation occurs in the last trimester of pregnancy, an increased desire for closeness with the husband is often felt (Chiota et al, 1976).

Factors which assist maternal attachment

Bodnar (1982) reports on a series of interviews with women whose pregnancies were classified as being 'at risk'. She found that when fears were decreased normal attachment behaviour generally continued.

One woman, who had had a previous anecephalic fetus found that she began to establish a relationship with her current baby after she had had an amniocentesis and found that this baby was not anecephalic. She said she talked inwardly to the baby and noticed whether it moved or whether it was having a quiet day. Another mother, who had had a previous stillbirth, did not relate to her baby at all until 39 weeks gestation. When she had an ultrasound she was told the baby was a boy and at this point she stated she really did believe now that there was a baby 'in there'. Following delivery she explained she had wanted to talk to the baby during pregnancy, as she had done with her first pregnancy, but was afraid of the sense of loss if something should go wrong again.

Another mother saw the photograph of the baby's head taken from the ultrasound. She was also shown the back and limbs on the screen. While she admitted she could not recognise these as identifiable parts of the baby, the explanation nevertheless gave her the concept of the reality of the newborn.

Nurses must assist mothers by providing information on the developing fetus and by using tests and test results to encourage attachment behaviours. At the same time sensitivity to the mother's current need for defense mechanisms to protect herself from loss is also essential. Mothers are receiving a multitude of signals from the medical profession which indicate that they should be sick, particularly once they are hospitalized. It is not surprising if alternative messages or measurements that indicate fetal well-being are not received (Bodnar, 1982). The need for reinforcement of all messages that indicate fetal well-being is essential and should be a planned element in nursing care of the high risk parent. Frequently the father is overlooked, yet he too needs explanation and reinforcement of the status and development of the fetus.

When the mother is admitted with a complication such as hypertension or antepartal bleeding she will tend to see the problem as hers. There is a potential threat to her as well as to the unborn baby. This increases her anxiety for she must be concerned both for herself and for the baby. In this vulnerable state the mother may cease all maternal-fetal attachment behaviours even when they have proceeded normally to this stage of pregnancy. Once again it is critical to ensure that the parents be provided with a full and careful explanation of the risks to mother and baby. All positive signs relative to the pregnancy should be reinforced.

Mothers who are experiencing an 'at risk' pregnancy have different expectations for their child-bearing experiences. Maternal-fetal attachment behaviours may be altered or delayed during the pregnancy and this may put the mother at risk for delayed postpartum attachment (Warrick, 1974; Cohen, 1979).

Nurses have the responsibility of exploring the psychological needs of mothers experiencing an at risk pregnancy. These mothers need an opportunity to express their thoughts in a non-judgmental atmosphere as a first step in their own exploration of their feelings. Nursing intervention includes activities to strengthen maternal support systems. Nursing actions include explanation of tests and procedures; continuation of normal prenatal classes; ensuring opportunities for maternal privacy and decreasing maternal powerlessness. To care for the 'at risk' mother the nurse needs an awareness of community resources and an awareness of family needs as well as counselling skills. In this way mothers and their families are assisted in coping with the stressful experience of a high risk pregnancy so that family bonds may be strengthened, rather than weakened, by the experience.

CONCLUSION

Physiological and psychological aspects of high risk pregnancy have been reviewed in this chapter. The need for continued monitoring and adequate supervision of mothers diagnosed as having a high risk pregnancy has been stressed. Caution must be exercised, however, in relation to women with normal pregnancy, who should not be subjected to unnecessary tests and procedures. The role of the nurse and/or midwife in providing support and guidance to high risk families is critical. In particular nurses and midwives can help identify the level of maternal-fetal attachment occurring in pregnancy. Measures that will encourage attachment behaviours have been described. A successful outcome in high risk pregnancy relies on a team approach and the parents must be considered a critical element in the team. The approach to investigation and treatment needs to be co-operative if a succcessful psychological, as well as physiological, outcome is to be attained.

REFERENCES

Avery G 1975 Neonatology, pathophysiology and management of the newborn. J. B. Lippincott, Philadelphia
Avery M E, Mead J 1959 Surface properties in relation to atelectasis and hyaline membrane disease. American Journal of Diseases of Children 97: 517–523
Battaglia F C 1970 Intrauterine growth retardation. American Journal of Obstetrics Gynaecology 106: 1103–1114
Behrman R 1977 Neonatal perinatal medicine, 2nd edn. Mosby, St Louis
Bibeau P, Perez R H 1980 Care of the intrauterine growth-retarded fetus. In: Butnarescu G F, Tillotson D M, Villareal P P (eds) Perinatal nursing volume 2: Reproductive risk. Wiley, New York.
Bodnar D 1982 The effect a physiologically at risk pregnancy has on the mother's self-esteem. Unpublished paper. Faculty of Nursing, University of Alberta, Edmonton
Bolsen B 1982 Question of risk still hovers over routine prenatal use of ultrasound. Journal of the American Medical Association 247: 2195–2197
Butnarescu G F, Tillotson D H, Villareal P P 1980 Perinatal nursing volume 2: Reproductive risk. Wiley, New York
Caplan G 1957 Psychological aspects of maternity care. American Journal of Public Health 47: 25–31
Chiota B J, Goolkasian P, Ladewig P 1976 Effects of separation from spouse on pregnancy, labour and delivery and the postpartum period. Journal of Obstetrics, Gynaecology and Neonatal Nursing 5: 21–23
Cohen R L 1979 Maladaptation to pregnancy. Seminars in Perinatology 3: 15–25
Colman A D 1969 Psychological state during first pregnancy. American Journal of Orthopsychiatry 39: 788–797
Colman A D, Colman L L 1973 Pregnancy as an altered state of consciousness. Birth and the Family 1: 7–11
Coleman C A 1981 Fetal movement counts an assessment tool. Journal of Nurse-Midwifery 26: 15–23
Cook N 1977 Intrauterine and extrauterine recognition and management of deviant fetal growth. Paediatric Clinics of North America 24: 431–451
Cranley M S 1979 Corinne: A mother at risk. American Journal of Nursing 79: 2117–2120
Evertson L R, Gauthier R J, Schiffrin B S, Paul R H 1979 Antepartum fetal heart rate testing I: Evaluation of the non-stress test. American Journal of Obstetrics Gynaecology 133: 29–33
Gauthier R J, Evertson L R, Paul R H 1979 Antepartum fetal heart rate testing II: Intrapartum fetal heart rate observation and newborn outcome following a positive contraction stress test. American Journal of Obstetrics and Gynaecology 133: 34–39
Garrett W J, Robinson D E 1970 Ultrasound in clinical obstetrics. Thomas, Springfield
Hartoon J C, Treuting E G 1981 Is noise a potential hazard to pregnancy? Occupational Health Nursing 33: 20–23
Health and Welfare Canada 1982 Sounding out on diagnostic ultrasound. Health and Welfare Canada, Ottawa
Hoffmaster J C 1978 Fetal movement as an indicator of fetal well-being. Perinatal Stress 6: 75
Hughey M J 1980 The ultrasound scan. In: Sarbargha R E (ed) Diagnostic

62   PERINATAL NURSING

ultrasound applied to obstetrics and gynaecology. Harper Row, New York
Ishii H, Yokoburi K 1960 Experimental studies on keratogenic activity on noise
    stimulation. Gunma Journal of Medical Science 9: 153–167
Mann L I, Tejani N, Weiss R 1974 Antenatal diagnosis and management of the small
    for gestational age fetus. American Journal of Obstetrics and Gynaecology 20:
    995–1004
Manning F A, Morrison I, Lange I R, Hartman C 1982 Antepartum determination of
    fetal health: composite biophysical profile scoring. Clinics in Perinatology 9:
    285–296
Miller H C, Hassaneim K M 1978 Socioeconomic factors in relation to growth in
    white infants. Directory of on-going research in smoking and health. U.S.
    Department of Health Education and Welfare
Peck T M 1980 Physicians' subjectivity in evaluating oxytocin challenge tests.
    Obstetrics and Gynaecology 56: 13–16. Saunders, Philadelphia
Penticuff J H 1982 Psychological implications in high-risk pregnancy. Nursing
    Clinics of North America 17: 69–78
Rayburn M D, Motley M E, Zuspan F P 1982 Conditions affecting non-stress test
    results. Obstetrics and Gynaecology 59: 490–503
Rayburn W F 1982 Antepartum fetal assessment. Clinics in Perinatology 9: 231–252.
    Saunders, Philadelphia
Rubin R 1961 Basic maternal behaviour. Nursing Outlook 9: 683–686
Rubin R 1975 Maternal tasks in pregnancy. Maternal Child Nursing Journal 4:
    143–153
Schiffrin B S 1982 The fetal monitoring polemic. Clinics in Perinatology 9: 399–408.
    Saunders, Philadelphia
Seeman M 1959 The meaning of alienation. American Sociological Review 24:
    783–791
Siegel M, Smookler H 1973 Fluctuating dental asymmetry and audiogenic stress.
    Growth 37: 35–39
Simpson W J A 1957 A preliminary report on cigarette smoking and the incidence of
    prematurity. American Journal Obstetrics and Gynaecology 73: 808–815
Snyder D J 1979 The high risk mother reviewed in relation to a holistic model of the
    childbearing experience. Journal of Obstetrics, Gynaecology and Neonatal Nursing
    8: 164–170
Strassman H T, Nochimson D J 1982 Determination of fetal maturity. Clinics in
    Perinatology 9: 297–312
Tejani N, Mann L I 1977 Diagnosis and management of the small for gestational age
    fetus. Clinical Obstetrics and Gynaecology 20: 943–955
Tejani N, Mann L I, Weiss R 1976 Antenatal diagnosis and management of the
    small-for-gestational-age fetus. Obstetrics and Gynaecology 47: 31–36
Verma W, Tejani N A, Chattergee S, Weiss R 1980 Screening for SGA by the rollover
    test. Obstetrics and Gynaecology 56: 591–594
Warrick L H 1974 An aspect of perinatal nursing: Support to the high risk mother.
    Presented at the American Nurses' Association Clinical Sessions, San Francisco.
    Appleton-Century-Crofts, New York
Weingold A B, Tan P J, O'Keefe J 1975 Oxytocin challenge test. American Journal
    Obstetrics and Gynaecology 123: 466–472
Williams L H, Maillot G, Hensley P A, 1981 Elevated amniotic fluid creatine.
    Obstetrics and Gynaecology 57: 28–34

Current practices in labour

INTRODUCTION

In medical and nursing practice we tend to be quicker to accept new ideas and techniques than to discard old ones, so that practices accumulate. The end result is unfortunate: an inevitably anxious mother comes to the hospital in early labour, prepared by excellent antenatal classes to expect one of the most happy and exciting episodes of her life, to be met by a frenzy of routines which at best may disappoint her and at worst frighten and humiliate her.

Many women have now come to see hospital delivery as something analogous to a chicken factory where they enter a conveyor to be plucked, cleaned out, trussed up and processed by practices whose relevance they cannot understand. And in the busiest hospitals dehumanization is increased by sheer lack of time to explain and reassure, so that we can no longer be surprised at the increasing groundswell of opinion that hospital delivery is an ordeal to be avoided in favour of delivery at home.

If the nursing profession believes, as it should, that a well equipped hospital is the safest place for delivery, then it has an obligation to continually assess its practices. Those that can be shown to contribute nothing must be discarded and new practices should be added only when it can be shown by thorough investigation that they are beneficial.

PREPARATION FOR NORMAL LABOUR

Childbirth has long since ceased to present a serious physical challenge to a healthy woman living in a civilized society; the dread of delivery a century ago, when maternal death was an everyday occurrence, has given way to confident expectation of a normal and happy outcome.

Antenatal care, beginning early in pregnancy, is widely advocated

63

not merely to detect those high risk conditions which may threaten the mother or her baby, and to ensure that she remains in good health, but also to maintain her confidence. This latter, more nebulous, aim may well be the more important. There is increasing evidence that women who are continually reassured particularly by regular contact with the same doctor or midwife, have better outcomes than those who do not have that support even though no active treatment may be given. For example women with twin pregnancies attending a supportive clinic where they see the same team each time do as well as those admitted to hospital for long periods of antenatal rest (O'Connor et al, 1981). The basis of this 'placebo' effect is not known, but whether it is due to a reduction in 'stress' resulting from increased confidence in their care, or some other mechanism, it is powerful and should not be underestimated.

Every woman probably experiences fear at some time during her pregnancy even when she is delighted at the prospect of motherhood. This anxiety is most often focused on the fear of having an abnormal child, but also relates to a fear of labour itself. It should not be forgotten that few women are immune to these anxieties; even doctors and midwives, although their knowledge and experiences give them an advantage, are prey to the same personal anxieties as any other pregnant woman. Because of these underlying fears, and above all because the pregnant woman is anxious to do whatever is best for her baby, the midwife is in a powerful position to play an effective educative role. Antenatal classes should reinforce the confidence-promoting activity of the clinic, and should also give the patient, *and her husband*, as much theorectical background as they need to understand the processes of pregnancy and delivery. A great deal of fear can be abolished by knowledge of what is going to happen.

Antenatal preparation for childbirth is practised by all good obstetric centres, but the extent of the preparation varies. Most antenatal classes teach the parents the elements of physiology of pregnancy, labour and infant feeding, and take this excellent opportunity with a receptive patient to instil the rudiments of sensible eating. Some classes emphasize exercises and include such elements as breast preparation, and preparation for childbearing reaches its ultimate expression in the techniques now attributed to the French obstetrician Lamaze. Books abound on the subjects of antenatal preparation and a detailed discussion would be out of place here; it is enough to say that while there can be little doubt that preparation is, in general, helpful, the importance or relevance of such components as exercises and controlled breathing techniques has never been tested. Preparation of the breasts by many manipulative techniques is certainly of no importance, and the wearing of the uncomfortable Waller's shields to correct poorly protractile nipples is valueless (Hytten & Baird, 1958).

It is the aim of psychoprophylaxis in pregnancy (the Lamaze system) to teach the mother how to be in total and confident control of her labour, preferably without the need for analgesia. One of the problems generated by such an approach is that the mother who fails to deliver easily or who feels impelled to ask for analgesia, may feel herself to be a failure and suffer guilt as a result. Her attendants in labour should be sufficiently knowledgeable and sensitive to antici- pate such a problem and explain the need for intervention in easily understood terms.

NORMAL LABOUR

It is important that the mother has clear guidelines about the appropriate point for her to come to hospital. She should be told that evidence of a show or ruptured membranes is sufficient reason to present herself in the labour ward whether or not she has contrac- tions, and that she should also come when her contractions are occurring regularly at intervals of 5 minutes or less. If she is in *any* doubt about being in labour she should come to hospital; it is better to be too early than to appear in advanced labour.

On arrival she should be seen by a midwife or doctor, her abdo- men examined, the fetal heart recorded, vaginal examination per- formed and, if amniotic fluid is draining, its colour noted. Routine recordings are begun of pulse rate, temperature, blood pressure, frequency and strength of uterine contractions and fetal heart rate.

Two time honoured activities are now questioned. These are perineal shave and evacuent enema. The original object of shaving and giving an enema was to admit a patient who was 'clean', with an empty 'clean' bowel and an unencumbered 'clean' perineum, to the delivery suite prior to parturition. It is a fact that patients find them distasteful; they take up midwives' time, which is an expensive resource; and the equipment and solutions used are expensive. In our hospital, Northwick Park Hospital and Clinical Research Cen- tre, we set out to establish the value of these procedures.

Shaving the perineum and pubic hair

Shaving the pubic area is a relatively modern practice and the early obstetric textbooks show no evidence of it. It probably arose in the early part of this century through the combination of two circumstances: the advent of aseptic surgical technique with its emphasis on a clean skin, and the arrival of the safety razor. It was also argued that the field of vision was improved by removing the hair.

There is no doubt that patients greatly dislike the procedure which is uncomfortable at best and can be moderately damaging in careless hands. Moreover they resent the prolonged irritation and discomfort of the hair growing again.

A series of 693 patients was studied (Romney, 1980) to determine the effect of pubic shaving on the incidence of infection in perineal wounds. A total of 228 patients had a complete shave, in 240 only the perineum was shaved and 225 were left unshaved. Shaving did not affect the incidence of infection and was associated with burning discomfort and itching in a high percentage of patients (Table 4.1). In addition there was frequent evidence of skin damage by shaving (Fig. 4.1). For these reasons we find it unnecessary to shave the perineum or pubic region, and never do more than clip particularly long perineal hair with scissors on admission.

Table 4.1 Incidence of perineal infection in 693 patients

Preparation	Infected	Not infected	Total
A. Unshaved	4	221	225
B. Complete shave	4	224	228
C. Perineal shave	7	233	240
Total	15	678	693

$P>0.50$, not significant

Enemas

The use of the enema is rooted in superstition and ritual and can be traced back to Egyptian, Roman and Greek practices. In present obstetric practice it is assumed that a bowel which is washed out before delivery will not contaminate the field during delivery, an advantage which is both bacteriological and aesthetic. It was also believed that stimulating the lower bowel also stimulated uterine action and speeded delivery. As with shaving, few patients enjoy it and most resent the discomfort of an enema.

Its value was examined in 274 women admitted for delivery of singleton infants; 149 were given an enema and 125 were not (Romney & Gordon, 1981).

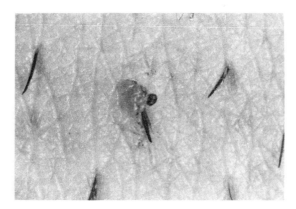

Fig. 4.1 High power photograph of skin after complete pubic shave. Note trauma in region of hair follicle and severe areas of bruising and haemorrhage. The changes were widespread over the whole area.

To the naked eye this seemed to be an atraumatic shave, but a magnified view shows multiple small abrasions. This supports the view of Kantor et al (1965) and demonstrates clearly that, even in skilled hands, a truly atraumatic shave is not possible.

The effect of faecal contamination, duration of labour, and infection in the baby are shown in Tables 4.2, 4.3 and 4.4. The incidence of gross faecal contamination was similar in the two groups, a surprising finding which suggests that the usual labour ward enema is relatively ineffective in cleaning out the lower bowel, and there was no influence on duration of labour. Seven newborn infants from each group showed evidence of infection, and bowel organisms were isolated from four in the no enema group and two in the enema group.

The overall evidence suggested that the pre-delivery enema offers no advantage. We now offer an enema only to women who have not had their bowels open for the past 24 hours, and to women who are found to have a loaded bowel on initial examination. There are also a very few women who believe they *should* have an enema, otherwise no bowel preparation is needed or given.

Use of electronic monitors

Monitoring in labour is part of the 'high technology' which many women now resent but which has nevertheless done much for the safety of the fetus. Here it is worth saying that the context in which the monitoring is done needs constant vigilance. For example to put

Table 4.2 Incidence of faecal contamination in labour. Combined series.

		% of women with no contamination	No. of women with no contamination	Women with contamination No. with grade			Total	Grand Total
				1	2	3		
			First stage					
Primigravid	Enema	84	51 } 95	7	1	2	10 } 19	61 } 114
	No enema	83	44	6	1	2	9	53
Parous	Enema	84	74 } 138	10	3	1	14 } 22	88 } 160
	No enema	89	64	6	1	1	8	72
Total	Enema	84	125 } 233	17	4	3	24 } 41	149 } 274
	No enema	86	108	12	2	3	17	125
			Second stage					
Primigravid	Enema	67	41 } 76	14	3	3	20 } 38	61 } 114
	No enema	66	35	11	2	5	18	53
Parous	Enema	66	58 } 100	17	9	4	30 } 60	88 } 160
	No enema	58	42	19	7	4	30	72
Total	Enema	66	99 } 176	31	12	7	50 } 98	149 } 274
	No enema	62	77	30	9	9	48	125

Significance of differences between untreated and control groups: first stage $x^2 = 0.17$, $P > .5$; second stage $x^2 = 0.52$, $P > 0.4$ (Student's test)

Assessment of results: The results in terms of faecal contamination were assessed on an arbitrary four-point scale: 0, clean (no contamination); 1, minimal faecal soiling but no formed motion or appreciable diarrhoea; 2, not more than two formed motions or episodes of diarrhoea; 3, frequent formed or fluid motions. We also considered the duration of labour and the incidence of infection in both mother and baby.

Table 4.3 Duration of labour in untreated (no enema) and control (enema) group of mothers (combined series)

	Duration of labour (hours)						Total
	≤4	−6	−8	−10	−12	>12	
			No enema				
Primiparae	14	12	7	9	5	6	53
Multiparae	36	11	7	15	2	1	72
Total	50	23	14	24	7	7	125
				Enema			
Primparae	14	8	11	12	6	10	61
Multiparae	40	20	14	8	4	2	88
Total	54	28	25	20	10	12	149

Table 4.4 Degrees of faecal contamination at delivery and sources of positive culture in 14 neonates in untreated and control groups with evidence of infection

Case no.	Grade of faecal contamination (0–3)		Site of positive swab	Organisms isolated
	1st stage	2nd stage		
				No enema
1	0	2	Eye	Escherichia coli, Streptococcus faecalis
2	0	3	Skin	Streptococcus faecalis
3	0	0	Nose	Escherichia coli, Streptococcus faecalis
4	0	0	Nose	Streptococcus faecalis
5	2	1	Umbilicus	Staphylococcus aureus
6	1	1	Eye	Staphylococcus epidermidis
7	0	1	Eye	Staphylococcus epidermidis
				Enema
8	0	2	MSU	Streptococcus faecalis
9	0	1	Skin	Coliforms, Proteus
10	1	1	Skin	Staphylococcus aureus
11	0	0	Eye	Staphylococcus aureus
12	0	0	Skin	Staphylococcus epidermidis
13	0	1	Eye	Staphylococcus aureus
14	0	1	Eye	Staphylococcus aureus

MSU = Midstream specimen of urine

an apprehensive patient in a room by herself, or even with her equally apprehensive husband, and to leave her for periods alone linked to a fetal monitor is as insensitive as it is foolish. Ideally no patient should be left at all without a midwife, but if that is not practicable then she should never be left for more than a few minutes; she should be constantly and cheerfully reassured, and the trace on the cardiotocograph should be explained to her frequently. The company of a cheerful midwife and constant reassurance are more important than a constant record of fetal heart rate. It is at least arguable that the monitor should be reserved for patients at risk and that little if anything will be lost and much gained if the role of the heart rate monitor is assumed by the midwife with a stethoscope. That proposition could at least be tested; there is no doubt it is what most patients would prefer.

Food and drinks

In most modern hospitals women in labour are forbidden food on the grounds that if the stomach is not empty then an emergency anaesthetic is dangerous because of the possibility of inhalation pneumonitis. Water is generally encouraged and it is now considered essential at least in Britain, for antacids such as magnesium trisilicate (15 ml) to be given regularly to eliminate the danger of Mendelson's syndrome. A word of caution should be given about the use of antacids; if any drugs are being given to the mother such as phenytoin to an epileptic, then absorption of that drug may be seriously reduced by complexation with antacid.

A word of warning is also necessary on the subject of ketonuria. If the labouring woman is allowed no food she is likely to become ketonaemic and the urine may be heavily charged with ketone bodies. Many hospitals react to that situation by infusing the mother with glucose solutions. Such a course of action is not only unnecessary but can be positively hazardous. Lawrence et al (1982) showed that although the infusion rapidly corrected the ketonaemia there was a significant rise in fetal plasma lactate and a fall in pH.

Positioning in labour and for delivery

A great deal of discussion both within the nursing profession and among the lay public now rages around the way a woman should behave in labour. Should she be confined to bed, or should she be allowed to walk about or adopt any position her restlessness might dictate? Should she deliver on her back in bed where most medical techniques and procedures can be best applied, or should she be allowed to find her own most comfortable position without regard to the convenience of conventional midwifery practices?

At the outset it is important to lay one persistent ghost that modern obstetrics has much to learn from the line followed 'instinctively' by primitive peoples. There is no such line as the detailed and scholarly compilation of anthropological data by Ploss et al (1935) makes clear. For example they detail the use of some 40 positions in labour, from lying supine to squatting, kneeling and even hanging from a tree. Those variations occur throughout the world with most of them represented in most countries and cultures. Moreover '... it is just among the peoples at the lowest stage of civilization that no uniform conduct of the woman with regard to the choice of position of the body for delivery has been observed.' As one anthropologist once observed, if the remote ancestry of mankind had instincts which, like the beaver, were dependent on structures in the brain, then these have long since ceased to exist and have given place to a freer and higher power of reasoning.

Variation in the practices surrounding labour extend far beyond the bodily position of the labouring woman. Women in many cultures choose to deliver their infants entirely alone, and among the original Incas of Peru: '... there was nobody who helped the women of any class whatever on this occasion, and if anyone attempted to assist them in childbirth, she was regarded as a witch rather than a midwife' (Garcillasso de la Vega, 1704, quoted by Ploss et al, 1935). Many other peoples deliver with a variety of assistants, and some deliver publicly, perhaps in a street. For those who did not deliver their baby by simply squatting on the ground there was a wide variety of accessory equipment ranging from vertical or horizontal poles, to blocks of wood, stones, or tubs and birth chairs or stools.

Finally there were and still are a great many mechanical and manual aids for delivery: bathing, anointing, massage, the application of pressure in various ways, and an astonishing number of devices to dilate the birth canal.

The huge proliferation of religious practices and of slimming diets attests to man's gullibility and it is easy for an articulate persuader to establish a belief. That is particularly true in the field of childbearing where pregnant women form an unusually susceptible group.

Herein lies a major problem. The doctrines of such evangalists as Leboyer are delivered in so emotive a style that while they may readily convince the impressionable pregnant woman, they cause an equal aversion among the more scientifically trained professionals. Both effects are perhaps unfortunate; a more moderate case might persuade the medical profession that there were at least some elements of sense in the suggestions and patients too would have been able to preserve a more balanced approach.

What we need to consider now, urgently but dispassionately, are the pros and cons of the different approaches. The increasingly vociferous group of women who demand the right to have their babies in any way they choose and to abandon such 'high technology' as fetal monitoring and epidural analgesia, deserve a reasoned answer.

What are the advantages, if any, of lying supine during delivery? Are there any demonstrable disadvantages? Does electronic fetal monitoring contribute more to the safety of the fetus than it detracts from the enjoyment of labour? And is pain relief useful, or dangerous or unnecessary? It is not yet possible to answer most of those questions in general and it may never be possible to answer them in relation to an individual.

CONTROVERSY REGARDING MANAGEMENT OF DELIVERY

Two of the most widely publicised 'gurus' in the field of labour management today are Frederick Leboyer and Michael Odent, both French. A brief discussion of their ideas will serve to illustrate the problems related to management of the delivery.

Leboyer's thesis is that the usual techniques associated with delivery, particularly in a modern hospital, are acts of psychological and physical violence to the newborn infant which do it permanent harm. No idea was better calculated to buttress the view of the growing army of women who had begun to rebel against what they saw as the unfeeling regimentation of hospital delivery. Leboyer's book *Birth without Violence* is an unashamedly emotional appeal to the lay public written in theatrical language which exploits every journalistic trick.

He describes the suffering of the newborn infant: 'The tragic expression, those tight-shut eyes, those puzzled eyebrows ... That howling mouth, that burrowing desperate head' and 'The whole creature is one jumping, twitching mass ... every inch of its body is crying out "Don't touch me" and at the same time pleading: "Don't leave me! Help me!" Has there ever been a more heart-rendering appeal? And yet this appeal — as old as birth itself — has been misunderstood, ignored, indeed unheard.'

Leboyer goes on to detail the assaults which are heaped on the infant, 'blinded' by strong lights, 'stunned' and 'deafened' by the 'world's uproar!', a 'thunderous explosion' of noises and voices, its skin assailed by rough and cold surfaces, and 'the burning sensation of air entering the lungs is the worst horror of all. Seared to its very depths the entire body quivers, shudders with horror, protests.' There is much more — the 'anguish' of being unsupported after its closely confined existence in the uterus, and then being left alone 'abandoned by everyone and everything, lost in a world as hostile as it is incomprehensible.' 'Unhappiness is so ingrained in most babies by this time that they hope for nothing else,' and 'remorse' that 'I am alive but I have killed my mother. I am here, but my mother is gone.' Stirring emotive words, and Leboyer's recipe for avoiding these horrors is logical. The baby should be delivered in subdued light into a peaceful quiet atmosphere, and placed face down ('*never on its back*') on the mother's bare abdomen. The cord should not be cut immediately: '*to sever the umbilicus [sic] when the child has scarcely left the mother's womb is an act of cruelty whose ill-effects are immeasurable. Birth without violence produces children who are strong, because they are free; without conflict.*'

Without careful research to evaluate such claims these assertions are open to question. The general public should understand that at this time there is no researched evidence which substantiates Leboyer's claims. Currently, there is no documented proof that shows that bright lights frighten a newborn infant, though many of the world's children throughout evolutionary time must have been delivered in sunlight. We also have no research to show whether the transition from the intrauterine noise levels recorded by Grimwade et al (1971) of up to 88 db (somewhere between the noise levels in a factory and in an underground train) to the 'world's uproar' in a normal delivery room deafens the baby. It is doubtful whether the claim that the handling the newborn receives after delivery causes it 'anguish' and 'remorse' can ever be substantiated.

Several comparative trails have been reported. Nelson et al (1980) in a small randomized study found no differences in maternal or newborn morbidity, in infant behaviour in the first hour of life, at 24 or 72 hours at 8 months, or in the mother's perception of her infant or the experience of delivery whether or not Leboyer's recommendations were followed. A somewhat larger study by Crystle et al (1980) in which infant morbidity was examined concluded that 'Leboyer's method of delivery does no harm and may well benefit initial family interactions and relationships.'

It would seem that stripped of its purple prose and preposterous claims, the Leboyer approach is sensible. Nobody could quarrel with the general proposition that it is preferable for a woman to be delivered in a serene atmosphere, and that she and her husband may gain from immediate loving contact with the baby; it is something which any well organized hospital could offer without sacrificing its conventional role. What is perhaps more dangerous is that some women may be so mesmerized by Leboyer's rhetoric, that if their baby should flinch when a bedpan is dropped inadvertently, they may believe it has incurred irreparable psychological damage.

An altogether more fundamental and complex challenge to conventional obstetric technique is the doctrine of Michael Odent. He has come to believe that women, when left to themselves, will adopt a whole range of positions in labour, squatting, kneeling or even standing in the second stage. He further believes that this behaviour is a 'regression' to a more primitive instinctive pattern and represents a refutation of the views of Lamaze:

> The importance we give to 'regression' emphasizes our radical opposition to the conventional 'psychoprophylaxis, which, on the contrary, has recourse to the stimulation of the upper cortex. The conventional 'psychoprophylaxis, is easily accepted in a world which requires a constant control of the emotions and of the body. O the contrary, the obstetrics we practice is chiefly dominated by the need to rehabilitate the emotional brain, the brain in tune with the body, the brain which controls the different aspects of the needs for survival. (A paper by Odent in the Bio-Energetic Journal, quoted by the NCT Journal New Generation, Vol. 1, page 81).

Many people in Britain watched a television programme on March 18th, 1982, of women delivering in Dr Odent's clinic. The impression was of labouring women and their attendants, mostly naked, in almost bare rooms, with the patient adopting all kinds of positions with support, usually from the husband. Conventional monitoring of any kind was absent and the perineum was left to its own devices. The claim that the system was ideal for labour with a breech presentation, illustrated by a squatting woman delivering a breech on to the floor, was somewhat undermined by the aside that the woman had required a Caesarean section some time later to deliver the second twin.

But as with Leboyer, it might be unwise to dismiss the whole of Odent's concepts on the basis of his own publicity. There may be some aspects of these ideas which are worth adopting and evidence exists for the advantages of delivery positions other than flat on the back.

If we are to meet the challenge from such ardent evangelists as Leboyer and Odent we must eliminate from our routines those things which are unnecessary and promote those aspects which they emphasize, *within the bounds of sensible and safe obstetrics.*

CREATING A LABOUR WARD/DELIVERY SUITE AMBIENCE

Perhaps the most universally important 'practice' is to establish the delivery suite as a pleasant reassuringly comfortable and friendly place to be. The expectant parents should become familiar with the environment where childbirth will occur and also meet the staff. The hardware they may encounter such as fetal monitoring equipment, inhalation analgesia machines, birth chairs and obstetric beds, should be demonstrated and explained in simple terms. The highly clinical hospital style delivery room, might be reserved for the more surgical circumstances and a less formal, more homely situation created for the normal process of childbirth.

Labour progress and delivery rooms should be comfortably furnished like an ordinary bedroom. The room should be tastefully decorated and colourful, with attractive curtains at the windows, and pictures on the walls. Soft background music can be piped from a central console and the woman in labour can choose to use this as a means of relaxation if she wishes.

Husband, boyfriend or other close friend or relative should be allowed to be present and support the woman throughout labour and delivery. Many husbands nowadays actively participate in providing effective emotional, psychological and physical support. The sharing markedly strengthens the loving links between them. Many women are anxious when separated from their close families, and particularly from their young children; there may be great advantage in having obstetric units with special family units where the parents, other children and selected relatives are allowed during labour and delivery. If the quiet serenity of a labour in the family circle can be carried through to delivery a lot of Leboyer's more useful ideas can be met without prejudice to effective medical care.

The adoption of some of Odent's more reasonable ideas is more difficult but feasible. For example there is usually no reason why a woman in normal first stage labour should not move about as she wishes. Many are restless and like to walk about or take up a variety of positions, but it is also a fact that many women, left to themselves, actually choose to lie on a bed. It has been claimed (Mendez-Bauer et al, 1976) that uterine contractions are of greater intensity in the upright position, and that labour is shorter (Diaz et al, 1978).

If the technological aids of fetal heart monitoring or oxytocin infusion are necessary they need not tie the patient down. The cardiotocogram can be monitored by remote telemetry, an expensive but perfectly satisfactory arrangement (Calvert et al, 1982) and there is no reason why oxytocin should not be given by one of the tiny portable battery driven syringes.

The position adopted by the mother in second stage is more contentious and the doctrines of Odent that she should be allowed to stand or squat or kneel or do whatever pleases her conflicts with the needs of the midwife who wants to see and guard the perineum and assist the delivery generally. Squatting in second stage, commonly adopted by many primitive peoples, carries a considerable anatomical advantage. Russell (1982) has shown that if the thighs are flexed and abducted the weight of the body causes a small separation at the lower end of the symphysis pubis with an outward movement of the innominate bones and a backward rotation of the sacrum. The net effect of these relatively small changes which have been observed radiologically is to increase the area of the *outlet* by 28% compared to the supine position. This is a very substantial advantage which may be worth the midwife making sacrifices of traditional practices.

It is possible, and the point should be studied, that delivery on a birth stool, or a modern birth chair (Fig. 4.2) might carry an equal advantage.

Our own experience with the birth chair is wholly favourable.

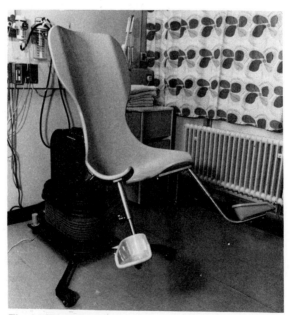

Fig. 4.2 The birth chair.

Women like it as they have less backache, they are better able to participate in the birth of their baby and can see it, and the midwife and doctor have excellent access.

Caldeyro-Barcia (1979) has claimed that the condition of the fetus is improved by delivery with the motther vertical on a birth chair, with a higher umbilical artery pO_2 and pH and a lower pCO_2. He attributes the difference both to more effective breathing by the mother and less interference with the blood supply to the uterus compared to the supine position.

ANALGESIA IN LABOUR

The administration of drugs for the relief of pain in labour is viewed by some as an unnecessary intervention by medical staff, causing unwanted loss of awareness and by others as a responsible attempt to relieve stress and anxiety.

Drugs administered to the mother inevitably cross the placenta to the fetus and the newborn infant is often less able to quickly excrete toxic substances or to transform them into non-toxic metabolites. Many mothers do not wish to be so affected by medication that they are distanced from what is going on in the delivery room and have a concern for the effect both on themselves and the baby during the early and vital period of their relationship with each other.

Nevertheless, doctors and midwives do have a clinical responsibility to relieve unacceptable levels of pain and stress. The aim must be to use as little medication as is compatible with individual need. Patient regulated intravenous pethidine enables a woman to use only as much as is required for comfort and she still retains participation in her own labour. Breathing and relaxation exercises can still be carried out.

If the woman's own control of events following good antenatal preparation and the judicious use of pethidine fails, the use of epidural anaesthesia should be discussed with her. This will remove her awareness of what is happening to her body, but will retain full mental alertness through the birth and introduction to her offspring.

THE USE OF EPISIOTOMY

Professional opinion is divided between those who use episiotomy routinely in order to prevent undue stretching and uncontrolled tearing of the perineal structures and those who use episiotomy only for a specific reason, such as delay in the second stage of labour giving rise to fetal distress. Immediate postpartum discomfort which persists and gives rise to dyspareunia are the main complaints from women who have had an episiotomy, but if it is properly performed and properly repaired as quickly as possible this should not be a problem. If the second stage of labour is progressing normally and there is no fetal distress and the perineal tissues are not overstretched it is doubtful that an episiotomy achieves anything more than additional discomfort for the mother. As in so many aspects of care in normal childbirth, the plea is for good clinical judgement related to the individual concerned.

THE THIRD STAGE OF LABOUR

In the period between 1930 and 1950, the third stage of labour was managed by masterly inactivity. The cord was only cut after pulsation had ceased and a resting period of at least 20 minutes was allowed following delivery of the baby. Manipulation of the uterus was regarded as a stimulation which would interfere with the normal process of placental separation and expulsion. The placenta was expelled by maternal effort when a suitable contraction occurred. It must be remembered that at that time there were many women of high parity in Western countries, and postpartum haemorrhage was a significant cause of maternal mortality and morbidity.

In the 1950s and '60s the now familiar Brandt-Andrews technique of controlled cord traction and the use of ergometrine was introduced, considerably reducing the severe postpartum haemorrhage. There have been side effects, not least of which are an increase in the occurrence of placental retention and an increase in secondary postpartum haemorrhage. It is now being questioned as to whether this technique which has life saving benefits in some cases, actually produces some abnormalities where none existed, in others. The problem with the third stage of labour in common with the first and second stage is that it can only be called normal retrospectively. The general health status, good nutrition and low parity of the women of Western countries today, may in themselves be responsible for a reduction in third stage complications.

In the United Kingdom the question is now being asked 'Should we relook at masterly inactivity in a proper controlled trial with Brandt-Andrews?' It is important to conduct such research as soon as possible before the best exponents of non active management have retired from service.

MOTHER'S RESPONSE TO BABY

Doctors and midwives working with couples through the transition to parenthood and during the actual birth process are ideally placed to make vital observations of the way parents react to their new babies and to note any problems which might inhibit the mother/baby bonding.

Specific kinds of maternal behaviour, such as nesting, retrieving, grooming and exploring are seen in many animal species; detailed and precise observations have clearly demonstrated that a definite pattern of behaviour also occurs in women. Human mothers appear to begin with a fingertip touching on the extremities of the infant, combined with a gentle stroking of the baby's face with the fingertips; the mother proceeds within the first 5 minutes to massaging by palm contact on the trunk. There is noticeable interest in the eyes of the infants when the mothers seek to establish an early eye to eye contact. It has been suggested that the eye to eye contact is one of the releasers of the maternal caretaking behaviour. Mothers tend to talk their babies using a high pitched voice. When speaking to other people in the room they revert to a normal voice tone.

After this initial stage of looking, touching and talking, mothers then express a wish to pick the baby up and hold it, maintaining an eye to eye contact. Following this there is a short interval when the interest seems to diminish. This phase of relative disinterest lasts for about 10–15 minutes. It is at this point that the baby may be put into its cot by the bed and the mother made comfortable following the delivery. Within the time this takes, interest reappears and the mother is then very receptive to holding her baby and actually putting it to the breast.

This pattern of behaviour following delivery seems to be important in the formation of the special mother/baby bonding process. Survival of the infant is not therefore left to chance; complex mechanisms appear to trigger maternal and infant behaviour in order to ensure the immediate care of the young offspring by its mother.

It should be noted and a record made when a mother does not respond in this way to her baby; if she does not touch, hold or examine him or talk in affectionate terms about him. Note should also be made when either parent reacts with hostility, and there should be concern when parents are disappointed about the sex of their baby and when they do not appear to be loving towards one another.

Acknowledgements

The authors wish to thank Professor F.E. Hytten for his advice, encouragement and help with this chapter.

REFERENCES

Caldeyro-Barcia R 1979 Physiological and psychological bases for the modern and humanized management of normal labour. In: Recent Progress in Perinatal Medicine and Prevention of Congenital Anomaly. Ministry of Health and Welfare, Tokyo, Japan, p 77–96

Calvert J P, Newcombe R G, Hibbard B H 1982 An assessment of radio-telemetry in the monitoring of labour. British Journal of Obstetrics and Gynaecology 89: 285–291

Crystle C D, Kegel E E, France L W, Brady G M, Olds R E 1980 The Leboyer method of delivery. An assessment of risk. Journal of Reproductive Medicine 25: 267–271

Diaz A G, Schwarcz R, Fescina R, Caldeyro-Barcia R 1978 Efectos de la posicion vertical materna sobre la evolucion del parto. Clinical Investigative Gynaecology Obstetrics 5: 101

Grimwade J, Walker D, Bartlett M et al 1971 Human fetal heart rate change and movement in response to sound and vibration. American Journal of Obstetrics and Gynaecology 109: 86–90

Hytten F E, Baird D 1958 The development of the nipple in pregnancy. Lancet i: 1201–1204

Kantor H I, Rember R, Tabio P, Buchanon R 1965 Value of shaving the pudendal perineal area in delivery preparation. Obstetrics and Gynaecology 25: 509–512

Lawrence G F, Brown J A, Parson R J, Cooke I D 1982 Feto-maternal consequences of high-dose glucose infusion during labour. British Journal of Obstetrics and Gynaecology 89: 27–32

Leboyer F 1975 Birth without violence. Wildwood House Ltd., London

Nelson N M 1980 A randomized clinical trial of the Leboyer approach to childbirth. New England Journal of Medicine 302: 655–660

Méndez-Bauer C, Arroyo J, Ménédex A, Salmean J, Manas J, Lavilla M, Martinez San Martin S, Villa-Elizaga I, Zamarriego Crespo J 1976 Effects of different maternal positions during labour. In: 5th European Congress of Perinatal Medicine, Uppsala, Sweden. Almqvist and Wiksell, Stockholm, p 233–237

O'Connor M C, Arias E, Royston J P, Dalrymple I J 1981 The merits of special antenatal care for twin pregnancies. British Journal of Obstetrics and Gynaecology 88: 222–230

Ploss H H, Bartels M, Bartels P 1935 Woman, An historical gynaecological and anthropological compendium, vol II. Heinemann, London

Romney M L 1980 Predelivery shaving: an unjustified assault? Journal of Obstetrics and Gynaecology 1: 33–35

Russell J C B 1982 The rationale of primitive delivery positions. British Journal of Obstetrics and Gynaecology 89: 712–715

Stewart P, Kennedy J H, Calder A A 1982 Spontaneous labour: when should the membranes be ruptured? British Journal of Obstetrics and Gynaecology 89: 39–43

Newborn care: An evaluation of silver nitrate prophylaxis

INTRODUCTION

The many factors which influence maternal responsiveness and the way in which infants develop emotionally, socially and intellectually are relevant both to the parents and to those with a professional interest and duty in maternal and infant health.

In our work we meet the new parents at a critical family-building time when they are changing and developing, and when they are most in need of advice and support. There must be a definite purpose to promote a positive experience of labour and of the baby's birth for both mother and father.

The results of research during the last two decades also indicate the importance of a gentle reception of the child at birth and of an early close contact between parents and their newborn (Leboyer, 1975). The experience of delivery and the first contact between the parents and the infant seem to influence their relationship and its further development. Research has shown that emotional bonds are developed in the mother already during pregnancy and in connection with the delivery, but that this sensitive biological process can be disturbed very easily during the first hours or days after birth.

It is often presumed in obstetric care that all the advanced technical resources and new methods will contribute to give the expectant mother and father a feeling of security. Nevertheless, some parents find that advanced maternity departments have an artificial and strange atmosphere.

During the 1970s research results, combined with health care debate, have influenced the practice and care routines in maternity clinics in my country, Sweden, as well as in most of the Western world.

Results of research indicate that several maternity and neonatal routines should be reconsidered. We need to examine critically the new and modern practices as well as those which have long been established by medical or care traditions and/or by state and municipal agencies. One of these practices is the use of silver nitrate for prophylactic eye care in the newborn.

SILVER NITRATE PROPHYLAXIS

Background

The practice of administering silver nitrate into the eyes of newborn infants to prevent gonococcal ophthalmia was introduced by the German obstetrician C.S.F. Credé in the early 1880s (Credé, 1881). At that time no effective treatment against eye infections existed, and the Credé prophylaxis proved to be one of the most successful measures in preventive medicine.

In the late 1800s *Neisseria gonorrhoeae*, discovered by A. Neisser in 1879, was recognised by several investigators as a major cause of neonatal ophthalmia. The fact that 20–80% of the children in institutions for the blind were there as the result of ophthalmia neonatorum was a matter of great concern. Credé (1881) reported that before the introduction of the silver nitrate prophylaxis, 10% of the infants born in the University Clinic of Leipzig had ophthalmia neonatorum and it was estimated that nearly all of these cases had a gonococcal conjunctivitis. After the Credé method had been introduced there was a rapid decrease in the incidence of gonococcal ophthalmia, from 10% to about 0.2% (Seedorff, 1960). Similar findings were reported in the United States for the same period, where a relationship between the introduction of Credé prophylaxis and a decrease in childhood blindness was noted (Barsam, 1966).

Medical statutes concerning Credé prophylaxis

Owing to the significant reduction in the frequency of gonococcal ophthalmia following treatment, instillation of 1–2% silver nitrate solution into the eyes of newborns was made obligatory during the first half of the twentieth century in most European countries and in most of the states of the U.S.A. At this time no effective alternative treatment of eye infections was available. Even following the advent of antibiotics in the 1940s, Credé prophylaxis has continued and its use is still regulated by statutes in many countries throughout the world, including the United States, Canada, Denmark, Iceland and Norway. In Sweden also a statute of the National Board of Health and Welfare instructs midwives to administer a 1% silver nitrate solution to the infant's eyes.

In some countries the procedure has been discontinued, for example in the United Kingdom (since the 1950s) and in the Netherlands (since 1981).

Credé method questioned — previous investigations

During the last three decades the need for Credé prophylaxis has been questioned by both professionals and parents in several countries. Many investigations have been carried out to evaluate the possible risk of discontinuing this treatment.

The results of a study undertaken in Toronto, Canada, were reported in 1955 by Ormsby. Among 2020 infants receiving no prophylaxis at birth there were five cases of gonococcal ophthalmia (0.25%), or eight times as many as in the control group given 1% silver nitrate solution. Another study was undertaken in 1958 by Seedorff in Copenhagen (at the request of the Danish National Health Service). In the department where no prophylaxis was given seven cases (7.6%) of gonococcal ophthalmia occurred, while in the control department where the usual Credé prophylaxis was administered there were none.

In 1955 the Board of Health in New York City permitted the use of various methods of prophylaxis against ophthalmia neonatorum. During the period 1956–1958 the frequency of gonococcal ophthalmia was studied among nearly half a million newborns. Greenberg & Vandow (1961) showed that among infants given no prophylaxis gonococcal ophthalmia occurred in 0.026% of babies, while in the groups given silver nitrate or physiological saline alone this figure was 0.007%. Among infants treated prophylactically with antibiotic ointments or solutions, 0.01% developed ophthalmiablennorrhoea, but there were no such cases in the group which had received intramuscular injections of penicillin. The investigators also showed that host and environmental factors were as important as the type of prophylaxis used. In areas with good maternal health records, no cases of ophthalmia occurred whether prophylaxis was used or not.

In many countries the discussion about the Credé method has become more intensified during the last few years, partly as a result of the attention paid to it by the mass media. The recent interest in parent-infant bonding has focused on the role of eye-to-eye contact between parents and their newborn.

The administration of silver nitrate is associated with pain and has long been abandoned in adult praxis. This painful instillation and the chemical conjunctivitis induced by Credé prophylaxis might interfere with the bonding process (Klaus & Kennell, 1976). Several authors have pointed out that eye contact plays an essential role in bonding and others have described the pleasure shown by new mothers when their infant begins to 'look' at them.

Butterfield et al have reported that paternal behaviour also seems to be affected by visual contact with the newborn. They found that infants with wide-open eyes received twice as much close looking and significantly more affectionate touching, and also for longer periods of time, than infants with closed eyes (Butterfield et al 1981).

Since the introduction of the Credé method the following changes have taken place with regard to the prevention, diagnosis and treatment of neonatal ophthalmia:

improved antenatal care has increased the possibility of diagnosing and treating gonnorhoeal infection during pregnancy

modern obstetric practices have diminished the duration of the birth process in cases of early rupture of the membranes, with a consequently reduced risk of ascending infections

in most developed countries births now take place in hospital and the infants are observed regularly during the first week of life by nurses and doctors

gonococcal ophthalmia can be readily cured by penicillin treatment.

Maternity care debate

The importance of psychological factors, such as bonding, during the first contact between parents and their newborn have been described by several authors (Klaus et al, 1975; Barnard, 1976). The mass media have also paid increased attention to behavioural and sociomedical factors affecting mother-infant dyads and their families.

During recent years some parents have said that delivery care in large maternity clinics is impersonal, artificial and institutional. At the same time we know that all the resources of the modern hospital are important and sometimes even necessary from the medical point of view, for the safety of the mother and infant may depend upon them. During the last ten years maternal and infant morbidity and mortality rates have fallen to a very low level in most of the Western world because of high standards of maternity care.

Human rights and ethical questions

The concept of human rights involves the observance of respect and reverence for the human being. The 'Convention for the Protection of Human Rights and Fundamental Freedoms' of the United Nations 1948 refers to a belief in fundamental human rights, in the dignity and value of the individual, and in equal rights.

The law concerning the Swedish Health Services (hospitals) is also based on respect for the patient's own wishes and on reverence for his or her integrity, as well as guaranteeing a high quality of care and paying due attention to the patient's need for safety and security. Further, according to this law the patient shall be informed about his state of health and about different methods of alternative care and treatment. Moreover, as far as possible the health and welfare care and services must be provided in co-operation with the patient. The health service regulations also point out the need for promotion of good contact between the patient and the health and hospital personnel.

According to the principal law of the Swedish Health Service (hospital), the Credé method in fact requires consent by the infant's legal representative, in most cases the mother, before the silver nitrate is given. If a mother rejects the prophylaxis, a conflict may arise between the mother's refusal and the duty of the midwife or staff to administer this treatment because of an earlier and still existing statute.

As a result of the intensive 'Credé controversy' of recent years, sometimes with referral to 'Human Rights', the Swedish National Board of Health and Welfare published a new circular concerning the prophylaxis in 1978. According to this instruction the National Board permits the midwife to withhold the prophylaxis in exceptional cases and under certain circumstances if this is the strict wish of the mother or parents. Comparable exemptions have also been permitted in Norway and Denmark.

The questions concerning the tradition-bound Credé prophylaxis have many ethical aspects. In several other countries opinions are expressed against this prophylaxis both among the public and the professionals. In spite of the stipulation in Health Service statutes that Credé prophylaxis be given, local or individual decisions are sometimes made to replace silver nitrate by, for example, penicillin or neomycin solutions, or an installation of lemon drops, or a decision may be made to omit prophylaxis altogether. These decisions are generally made on an individual basis and are in contravention of the existing law.

EVALUATION OF CREDÉ PROPHYLAXIS

Aims of the study

The principal aim of this investigation was to find out whether Credé prophylaxis had mainly positive or mainly negative physiological consequences. A further aim was to investigate the influence of Credé prophylaxis and some other care routines on the early bonding process between mothers and their newborns and to examine possible long-term effects of such treatments. Epidemiological aspects of some venereal diseases were also examined.

General study design

Mother-infants and main methodology

The investigation comprised more than 1000 consecutive mothers and their newborn infants, delivered at the Karolinska Hospital, Stockholm in 1978.

The study examined the frequency of maternal gonococcal and Chlamydial infection (epidemiological study); the pain reactions and the frequency of signs of conjunctivitis following different kinds of eye prophylaxis, i.e. 1% silver nitrate, 10% Hexarginum (a less irritating silver compound) or physiological saline (as placebo) in a randomized double-blind study. The in vitro antibacterial effects of silver nitrate and of Hexarginum were also studied.

Furthermore, behavioural studies were performed, one in order to examine the effects of eye prophylaxis on visual alertness, and one to study the effects on mother-infant relationship. At 3 and 6 months postpartum interviews and questionnaires, respectively, were answered by mothers in a follow-up study (Table 5.1).

Table 5.1 Number of mother-infant pairs participating in different studies of the Credé investigation

Study	No.
Epidemiological study	1027
Effects on visual alertness	39
Effects on mother-infant relationship	65
Long-term influences (follow-up)	136

For the present Credé investigation a dispensation was received from the statute of the Swedish National Board of Health and Welfare and the project was approved by an Ethical Committee.

Information to and consent of the mothers/parents

During the study period, informed consent for participation in the study was obtained from all mothers/parents when they arrived in the delivery ward. They were told by the midwives that the purpose was to reconsider the practice of silver nitrate prophylaxis; that a randomized series of numbered and non-returnable bottles would be used for eye prophylaxis; of these bottles, 20% contained silver nitrate solution, 40% contained Hexarginum and 40% contained physiological saline. Prophylaxis was given about 2 hours post-partum.

During the total study period no parents refused to participate. The high compliance may have been due to the current consumer concern about silver nitrate prophylaxis (Table 5.2).

Table 5.2 Assignment of newborns to different prophylactic groups

	n
Silver nitrate 1%	105
Hexarginum 10%	225
Placebo (physiological saline)	214
No prophylaxis*	83

*children born after Caesarean section

Routines in delivery room and maternity ward

During the study period the delivery and the care routines were as follows: The father was usually present at labour and delivery. When analgesia was administered it usually consisted of 50–100 mg of pethidine plus pudendal block. Epidural analgesia was given in 14% of the deliveries. Immediately following birth the baby, naked or wrapped in a sheet was placed on the mother's abdomen and was usually left there for 20-30 minutes. The infant was then taken away for a short while for weighing, measuring, and dressing. Afterwards the mother, father and infant were left in private in the delivery room for about two hours. The ophthalmic prophylaxis was then given, and the mother and child were taken to the maternity ward. Here the rooms have either two or four beds. Rooming-in during the daytime was generally practised during the 5–7-day hospital stay.

Daily inspection of infants' eyes

During the stay in the maternity ward the children's eyes were inspected daily, between 8 and 11 a.m. Swelling of the eyelids, redness of the conjunctiva and secretion were recorded. Neither the mothers nor the observers knew to which prophylactic group the infants belonged (Table 5.3).

Table 5.3 Number of mothers and infants participating in different parts of the Credé investigation

	n
Mothers	
Culture for gonorrhoea from urethra, cervix, and rectum	1027
Culture for Chlamydia from urethra and cervix	165
Infants	
Registration of pain reaction at administration eye drops	810
Registration of conjunctivitis/irritation by daily observation	627
Bacterial culture of newborns with conjunctivitis	156
Culture for Chlamydia from eyes	
subsample	250
infants with longlasting conjunctivitis	15

Effects on visual alertness

The sample for this study comprised 39 infants previously randomized to the three prophylactic groups and observed on the second

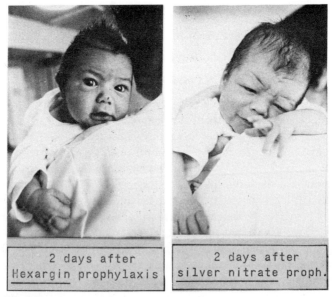

2 days after
Hexargin prophylaxis

2 days after
silver nitrate proph.

Fig. 5.1

and fourth days after birth.

Observations of the infants' visual alertness were made according to a method described by Korner & Thoman (1970), which provides 'vestibular stimulation' (infants were lifted from a supine position to the attendant's shoulder). The observer did not know to which prophylactic group the infants belonged.

Effects on mother-infant relationship

The purpose of this work was to compare the effects on mother-infant interaction and on maternal attitudes of silver nitrate and Hexarginum instilled prophylactically into the eyes of newborn infants.

A directional hypothesis for the study was as follows: The chemical conjunctivitis induced by silver nitrate will negatively influence the maternal attempts to make eye contact, and en face behaviour even after the conjunctivitis has disappeared.

The sample consisted of 65 mother-infant pairs previously randomized to silver nitrate and Hexarginum groups in a double-blind fashion. Observations were done between 8 and 10 a.m. on the fourth or fifth day after birth during the mother's care of the infant and during breast-feeding. An interview followed the last observation session and a second interview was conducted by telephone 6–8 weeks later.

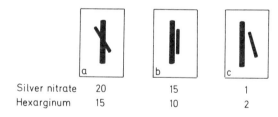

	a	b	c
Silver nitrate	20	15	1
Hexarginum	15	10	2

Fig. 5.2 Position of mother-infant during breast-feeding
a = mother sitting
b + c = mother lying down

Follow-up study

A follow-up study comprised 136 consecutive, healthy primi- and multiparous mothers and their healthy infants. The mothers were asked to take part in an interview by telephone 3–3½ months postpartum and to answer a questionnaire 6 months postpartum.

The interview and the questionnaire comprised questions concerning the experiences of the delivery itself, the first contact with the newborn infant and several other events around birth and the following months. Some questions were also asked about possible local side effects of the prophylactic drops during the weeks after birth. All 136 mothers who were asked to be interviewed participated in the study, and 96% of them answered the questionnaire. Neither the mothers nor the investigators knew to which prophylactic group the infants belonged.

MAIN OUTCOMES OF THE STUDY

Clinical findings

In the present population maternal gonococcal infection was observed in $\frac{1}{1027}$ women and maternal Chlamydia infection in $\frac{1}{165}$ women of the sub-sample; in both instances the infections were clinically asymptomatic. There were no cases of gonococcal ophthalmia, but among 15 infants who showed a long-lasting conjunctival irritation Chlamydia was isolated in two (Table 5.4).

Table 5.4 Occurrence of gonorrhoea and Chlamydia infections in healthy mothers during delivery, in healthy newborns, and in newborns with conjunctival secretion

	Culture	No. examined	No. with proven infections
Mothers before delivery	Gonorrhoea	1027	1
	Chlamydia	165	1
Healthy infants	Chlamydia	250	0
Infants with conjunctival secretion during the postpartum week	Gonorrhoea	156	0
Infants with longstanding conjunctival secretion 12–15 days postpartum	Chlamydia	15	2

The reaction of the newborn to silver nitrate was considerably stronger than that to Hexarginum and physiological saline with respect to pain and other side effects.

The observation of pain reactions (crying and averting movements) showed that silver nitrate induced significantly more violent reactions ($p < 0.002$) than Hexarginum and saline. The frequency of crying was significantly higher for girls compared with boys. Conjunctivitis was much more common in the Credé group than in the two other groups. Almost 40% of the silver nitrate infants had a purulent secretion during days 1–3, but only 2% of the Hexarginum and the saline groups (p<0.001) as shown in Figure 5.3.

Behavioural findings

Effects on visual alertness

Infants in the silver nitrate group showed less alertness and scanning behaviour on the second day postpartum than did infants in the Hexarginum and physiological saline groups. These differences were significant only between the silver nitrate and Hexarginum groups (p<0.05). On the fourth day postpartum these differences had disappeared.

There were no differences in scores of visual alertness between girls and boys, nor between infants of primiparae and multiparae.

Although crying was not included as an item in the visual behaviour score, it was observed that when lifting the crying infants

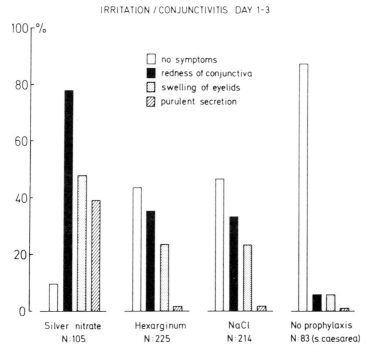

Fig. 5.3 Occurence of irritation or conjunctivitis on days 1–3 in 627 children given different types of prophylaxis

from table to shoulder, almost of them stopped irrespective of prophylaxis group. This was true for both day 2 and day 4 observations.

Effects on mother-infant relationship

During the observation of the mother's care of the infant (changing diapers and washing the baby) no significant differences in maternal or infant behaviour were found between the two prophylactic groups. During breast-feeding mothers of silver nitrate infants showed significantly less attempts to make eye contact, and 'en face' behaviour with their infants than did mothers of the Hexarginum group (p<0.05) (Table 5.5).

Table 5.5 The variables in Observation II (breast-feeding). Twenty periods registered.

Variable	Mean score		Standard deviation	
	Silver nitrate	Hexarginum	Silver nitrate	Hexarginum
	n = 36	n = 27	n = 36	n = 27
Maternal behaviour				
holding infant	17.1	14.0	6.7	8.8
attempt to eye contact*	1.1	2.3	2.5	2.9
looking 'en face'*	0.5	1.5	1.6	2.3
talking to infant	7.8	10.0	5.8	6.6
encompassing	11.9	8.3	9.0	9.0
affectionate touch love (ATL)	9.0	8.3	5.2	6.0
looking at infant	18.5	18.4	3.8	3.8
smiling at infant	2.4	2.0	3.7	4.0
breast-feeding	16.1	15.7	3.5	4.8
close contact	18.9	17.6	4.6	6.3
empathy (scale 1–5)	3.4	3.2	1.1	1.0
Child behaviour				
opened eyes	9.6	11.5	6.1	7.3
closed eyes	10.4	8.5	5.9	7.2

*p<0.05; Z-test of a directional hypothesis. Observed Z = 1.72 and 1.94 respectively. Critical value = 1.64 on the 5% level.

Stress factors, for example, a complicated delivery (vacuum extraction, cervical rupture, haemorrhage >600 ml) seemed to potenitate the mother-infant eye contact (p>0.02) (Fig. 5.4).

Maternal attitudes towards the child, their delivery and their postpartum care, as expressed 4 days and 6 weeks after delivery, did not differ between the groups. The frequency of breast-feeding at 6 weeks was similar.

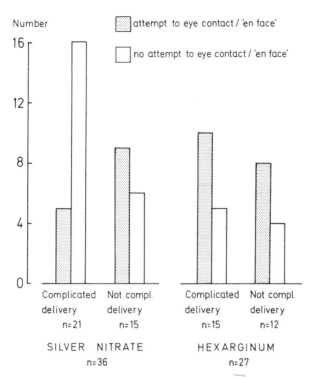

Fig. 5.4 Mothers attempt to make eye contact and 'en face' behaviour during breast-feeding in relation to complicated delivery (vacuum extraction, cervical rupture, haemorrhage 600 ml) (p<0.02, Fisher's exact test: 6.61)

Follow-up study

8–10 weeks postpartum, when nearly all eye irritation had disappeared in the physiological saline group, it was found that 21% of the silver nitrate group and 12% of the Hexarginum group still had persistent eye irritation.

The mothers also estimated the age at which the infants were able to focus and follow an object with their eyes. The average estimated age was 4.4 weeks (range 1–10 weeks). There were no significant differences between the groups nor between the estimations of primiparous and multiparous mothers.

The mothers' answers concerning their perceptions of the delivery, their first contact with their newborns and some other selected events at the time of birth and during the following months were analyzed. Since there were no significant differences between the three prophylactic groups regarding any studied relevant variable, the data were combined for the total group (n = 136). This analysis showed that 32% of full-term infants had been separated from their mothers and most of them had been placed in an incubator within 10 minutes of birth. Episiotomy had been performed in 40% (primiparas 58% and multiparas 26%). At 3 months a frequency of 24% of newborns was reported as having a colicky cry/pain for 3–4 hours a day during 4 or more weeks.

When the colic group of 32 infants was compared with the remaining 104 infants, significant differences between the groups were found for the following variables: 'separating the infant from the mother within 10 minutes postpartum' (p<0.001) and 'placing the infant in an incubator within 10 minutes postpartum' (p<0.01) (Table 5.6). This will be discussed further under 'Importance of maternal and neonatal period'.

Table 5.6 Events during labour and delivery in the group of infants reported by their mothers as having colicky cry/pain (n = 32 or 24% of the total group), compared with the remaining 104 infants. Interview 3 months postpartum. s 17

Variable	Infants with colicky cry/pain n = 32		Infants without colicky cry/pain n = 104		Significance
	No.	%	No.	%	
Epidural analgesia	10	31	24	23	NS
Episiotomy	17	53	37	36	NS
Vacuum extraction	6	19	18	17	NS
Infant separated from mother within 10 minutes postpartum	20	62	24	23	<0.001
Infant also placed in incubator 10 minutes postpartum	16	50	22	21	<0.01

POSITIVE AND NEGATIVE CONSEQUENCES OF CREDÉ PROPHYLAXIS

At the start of the present study on Credé prophylaxis the principal question was: Does the Credé method have mainly positive or mainly negative consequences?

Positive consequences

The Credé method of prophylaxis was an extremely important discovery at a time when no effective treatment against gonococcal ophthalmia was available. After the introduction of silver nitrate prophylaxis there was a rapid fall in the incidence of this disease. The following positive factors must be emphasized:

It has been one of the most important successes in preventive medicine
It has prevented eye damage and blindness in numerous human beings
It is inexpensive and involves a simple technique.

Negative consequences

From this investigation of the question of Credé prophylaxis from a somatic, bacteriological and behavioural point of view and from reports in the literature the following conclusions have been drawn concerning the immediate negative consequences:

It is painful (causing the infants to close their eyes immediately) and consequently disrupting to the gentle reception of the child following birth
It has a solely local, temporary effect (the oro-pharynx can become colonized during the passage through the birth canal)
It does not give a 100% guarantee of prevention
It frequently causes swelling, redness and purulent secretion in the eyes
Its side effect (purulent conjunctivitis) can hide a genuine gono-coccal infection, which may be mistaken for a chemical one with a consequent delay of therapy
The conjunctivitis frequently disturbs early, spontaneous eye contact of the parents with their newborn child.

In addition to the immediate negative consequences, the effects on the mother-infant relationship during the maternity stay must be mentioned. In this study it was found that mothers of infants in the Credé group showed fewer attempts to make eye contact and to have 'en face' behaviour than did mothers in the Hexarginum treatment group.

The rather moderate differences between the two groups, found with the methods of observation that were used, were somewhat unexpected, in view of the stated importance of early eye-to-eye contact between parents and infant. The results were especially surprising when one takes into account the interest mothers often express regarding their infants' eyes. The fact that silver nitrate, which induced chemical conjunctivitis, had so little obvious effect on maternal behaviour, might be explained by the special care routines practised in our hospital, which have also been introduced in many delivery wards in recent years. For example, the postponement of the Credé prophylaxis for 1–2 hours, and the immediate postnatal close body contact and 'rooming-in' in the maternity ward, may have contributed to the mother-infant bonding that was observed to have occurred (Korner & Grobstein, 1966; Klaus et al, 1972; Huesgen, 1979).

It is possible that if these factors, which are said to promote bonding, had not been present, the differences between the groups might have been greater. This assumption is supported by the observation that the negative effect of Credé prophylaxis was more pronounced among the women with complicated deliveries than among those with normal deliveries. These women had not had early body contact with their newborn. Thus, Credé prophylaxis seems to be one of several factors which contributes to a cumulative negative effect.

Necessity of prevention against gonococcal ophthalmia

In view of the potentially negative consequences of Credé prophylaxis, the question is raised as to the need for preventive measures in countries with good health records. Greenberg & Vandow (1961) showed that host and environmental factors were more important in the prevention of gonococcal ophthalmia, than the type of prophylaxis given. In areas with high medical and health standards no cases of ophthalmia occurred whether prophylaxis was used or not. The risk of blindness due to untreated gonococcal ophthalmia would thus be very low in developed countries, where antibiotics are also readily available to institute prompt treatment if required. While Credé prophylaxis has not been used in Britain since the 1950s, there have been no reports of blindness from gonococcal ophthalmia (Schofield & Shanks, 1971) which would offer support to this assumption.

Nevertheless, in developing countries where no prophylaxis against gonococcal ophthalmia exists, there may well be a need for some prophylaxis and silver nitrate is both cheap and convenient. However, in developed countries and/or parts of societies which today use the traditional Credé method, an alternative is needed. In these situations Hexarginum may be an alternative to gonococcal prophylaxis, since it is almost as effective as silver nitrate in killing gonococcus in vitro (Moberg Kallings & Wahlberg, 1982), yet, at the same time, Hexarginum, was found to result in fewer side effects than the silver nitrate solution.

If statutes on Credé prophylaxis are repealed it is of the utmost importance that every case of conjunctivitis with purulent discharge, whether occurring during the stay in hospital or after coming home, be investigated without delay. The staff and the parents should be instructed that a sample of the discharge from the eye must be taken immediately for direct microscopic examination and for culture.

If silver nitrate is replaced by Hexarginum, a similar policy is recommended. The present findings suggest that in either case, that is without treatment or with the use of Hexarginum, a purulent discharge will appear in some 2% of the newborns, the great majority of non-gonococcal origin. With such small numbers the burden on the laboratory will thus not be great.

Instances of neonatal gonococcal ophthalmia seem to be reported rarely today in countries with good health records. A review of the existing regulations concerning compulsory notifications is recommended whether the prophylaxis is continued or not. Compulsory notification of neonatal Chlamydia should be considered.

IMPORTANCE OF MATERNAL AND NEONATAL PERIOD

Research has shown that emotional bonds develop between the mother and infant during the course of pregnancy and during labour and delivery, but that this sensitive process can be disturbed very easily during the first hours or days of the postpartum period (Klaus et al, 1975; de Chateau & Wilberg, 1977). During the 1970s results from research in bonding resulted in health care debates that influenced the practice and care routines in many maternity clinics.

Some effects of routines around the birth of the newborn

Some modes of delivery combined with the effects of analgesia and anesthesia, some measures used in the immediate care of the infant and some nursing care routines in maternity and neonatal wards, involve separation of the mother from the newborn. This separation can give rise to disturbances during the early bonding process, a period where there is an active exchange of signals between mother and infant.

Early separation has been related to a high frequency of disturbances in infant behaviour during the first year of life, anxiety during the night, crying or screaming, colicky cry/pain, vomiting, and low weight gain. If the very early period of infancy really is of such great importance as different investigations indicate, there are reasons to search more thoroughly for possible causal connections between such disturbances and today's care routines in delivery, maternity and neonatal wards. We must find out what routines are favourable or unfavourable to infants and to the further development of their relations with their parents and family and urbanized society.

At the same time that convincing research findings have been presented that identify the significance of bonding, a highly technological and mechanical form of care has been developed. Active management of labour, advanced modes of analgesia and hormone therapy, for example, involve a risk that the infant will not be born in accordance with human nature. One extreme example of active management, is the idea of delivering infants during 'office time' using amniotomy (artificial rupture of membranes) followed by uterine stimulation. Another example is the high frequency of episiotomy, which often causes the infant to be delivered or 'forced out' of the birth canal too rapidly. Perhaps the birth itself should be handled in a more careful and cautious way, allowing, if possible, a natural development of labour and delivery, where the infant can be born in accordance with its own rhythm (Leboyer, 1975).

Also for the mothers the episiotomy is often experienced as something abnormal. Many women experience discomfort and problems for a long time postpartum. The episiotomy rate has increased rapidly as modern obstetric routines have developed. The question of the impact on the infant of analgesics taken at this time in relation to the concentration of drugs expressed through the breast milk has also been raised.

Possibly many of the events such as the high rate of episiotomy, the separation of the baby from the mother immediately after birth, and incubator care could be reduced, without harm to mother or baby. Perhaps the frequently used routine of gastric evacuation in newborns by intubation should be researched to see if it serves any useful purpose.

Findings related to mothers and infants in follow-up study

A follow-up study of the mothers who received Credé prophylaxis was undertaken and was of a descriptive nature. While adding long-term data on newborn behaviour related to Credé prophylaxis information was also sought on the mothers' experiences of events around the time of birth and in the following months.

This study showed that 32% of the 136 infants were separated from their parents and most of these 32% were placed in an incubator within 10 minutes after birth. A majority of the mothers, whose infants were separated from them at birth, have described their unforgettable and very positive experience of the brief contact they had with their newborn before the baby was taken away from them. Many of them have also expressed feelings of dismay, disappointment and total helplessness about their separation from their newborn. Unfortunately, we could not ask the infants about their feelings relating to the separation.

It must be asked: Do we really need this high rate of separation and incubator care for full-term infants? How often is the decision made because of a concern for the infant's temperature fluctuation? Gardner (1979) reports that when the mother is used as an incubator, after delivery there is no difference in body temperature between infants given mother-contact and infants that receive incubator treatment. In one group nude infants were held next to their mothers' bodies, and their decreases in temperature were compared with those of a second group of infants, who were kept in a Kreisselman bed. After 15 minutes both groups had identical temperatures of 36.7°C, which was well above the acceptable minimum body temperature of 36.1°C.

In this follow-up study 24% of the infants were reported by their mothers to have colicky cry/pain. Because this seemed to be a high percentage the frequencies of some potentially associated variables were examined (Table 5.5). When the colic group was compared with the no-colic group, the variable of early separation was found to be related to the incidence of colic.

Colicky crying is one of the most common complaints during the first few months of life. Colic is often a major cause of family disturbances during this period, and one can presume it is more commonly seen in vulnerable families and that vulnerability may be related to separation. It is a symptom of great significance. The possibility that it may be iatrogenic cannot be ignored and should be investigated further. Meanwhile, it is important to examine the necessity of the separation routines.

The findings concerning colic in the present study must, however, be intepreted with caution and have to be reconfirmed in a further controlled investigation. Other authors have also explored the suggestion that the ultimate cause of colic may be maternal anxiety (Paradise, 1966; O'Donovan, 1980).

Perhaps we need to ask ourselves: How do we meet and treat the new human beings during the birth process in our modern maternity hospitals? Do we contribute to disturbing the sensitive bonding process by a too artificial and strained beginning to life, and do we produce anxiety in both the mother and her baby by our ambition to do our best?

Reverence for the gift of life and respect for the human being

In the laws governing the Swedish Health Service (hospitals) there is a stipulation that respect should be paid, as far as possible, to the liberty and equality of human beings and to the individual's wishes, a consideration which belongs under the heading of Human Rights. Many nursing theories also point out that care and cure should be a 'helping service', rendered with compassion, skill and understanding to those in need of care, advice and confidence in the area of health.

The philosophy of health care personnel concerning their central purpose is important for the quality of the care given. We must believe in certain values and express them by our actions and attitudes towards our patients. Wiedenbach (1970) identifies three essential components of this philosophy:

a reverence for the gift of life
respect for the dignity, value, autonomy and individuality of each human being
a resolution to act dynamically in accordance with one's own beliefs.

Within the field of maternal newborn-care there is a need for nurses to evaluate current practices and to determine the benefits and determinants of each one in terms of the immediate and long-term consequences for both parents and newborn. As nurses we can then respond to parental concerns and aid them in making informed decisions in relation to desirable procedures for delivery and newborn care.

REFERENCES

Barnard K 1976 The process of maternal acceptance. In: The first week of neonatal life. Report from the 1st Maternal-Infant Life Conference, Oshkosh, Wisconsin, p 79–83
Barsam P C 1966 Specific prophylaxis of gonorrhoeal ophthalmia neonatorum. A review. The New England Journal of Medicine 274: 731–734
Butterfield P M, Einde R N, Platt B B 1978 Effect of silver nitrate on initial visual behaviour. American Journal of Diseases of Children 132: 426

Butterfield P M, Einde R N, Svedja M J 1981 Does the early application of silver nitrate impair maternal attachment? Pediatrics 67: 737–738

Credé C S F 1881 Die Verhütung der Augenzundung der Neugeborenen. Archives Gynacology 17: 50–53

de Chateau P, Wiberg B 1977 Long-term effect on mother-infant behaviour of extra contact during the first hour post partum. II. A follow-up at three months. Acta Paediatrica Scandinavica, 66: 145–151

Gardner S 1979 The mother as incubator — after delivery. Journal of Obstetrics Gynaecology Neonatal Nursing 8: 174–176

Greenberg M, Vandow J E 1961 Ophthalmia neonatorum: Evaluation of different methods of prophylaxis in New York City. American Journal of Public Health 51: 836–845

Huesgen Curry MA 1979 Contact during the first hour with the wrapped or naked newborn: Effect on maternal attachment behaviours at 36 hours and three months. Birth and the Family Journal 6: 227–235

Klaus H M, Jerauld R, Kreger N C, McAlpine W, Steffa M, Kennell J H 1972 Maternal attachment. Importance of the first postpartum days. The New England Journal of Medicine 286: 460–468

Klaus M H, Kennell J H 1976 Maternal-infant bonding. Mosby, St Louis p 70–78, 95

Klaus M H, Trause M A, Kennell J H 1975 Does human maternal behaviour after delivery show a characteristic pattern? In: Porter E, O'Connor M (eds) Ciba Foundation Symposium 23 (New Series). Elsevier, Amsterdam, p 69–85

Korner A F, Grobstein R 1966 Visual alertness as related to soothing in neonates. Implications for maternal stimulation and early deprivation. Child Development 37: 867–876

Korner A F, Thoman E B 1970 Visual alertness in neonates as evoked by maternal care. Journal of Experimental Child Psychology 10: 67–78

Leboyer F 1975 Birth without violence. Alfred A Knopf (ed), New York

Moberg Kallings I, Wahlberg V 1982 Reconsideration of Credé prophylaxis. II: Antibacterial effects of silver nitrate as used for Credé prophylaxis and of a colloidal silver compound — Hexarginum. Acta Paediatrica Scandinavica, Supplement 295, p 37–42

O'Donovan J C 1980 Infantile colic, or what to do until the fourth month comes. Comprehensive Therapy 6: 9–12

Ormsby H L 1955 Ophthalmia neonatorum. Canadian Medical Association Journal 72: 576–580

Paradise J L 1966 Maternal and other factors in the etiology of infantile colic. Journal of the American Medical Association 197: 191–197

Schofield R A, Shanks R H 1971 Gonococcal ophthalmia neonatorum despite treatment with antibacterial eye-drops. British Medical Journal 1: 257–259

Seedorff H H 1960 Is prophylactic treatment of the eyes of the newborn infants still necessary? Danish Medical Bulletin 7: 128–131

Wahlberg V 1982 Reconsideration of Credé prophylaxis. A study of maternity and neonatal care. Medical dissertation. (Co-authors: Lundh W, Moberg Kallings I, Winberg J.) Acta Paediatrica Scandinavica, Supplement 295

Wiedenbach E 1970 Nurses' wisdom in nursing theory. American Journal of Nursing 70: 113–134

Issues in the care of the low birthweight infant

INTRODUCTION

A number of issues currently exist in the care of the low birthweight infant. Ethical issues related to the preservation of life, the choice of candidates for scarce medical resources, and research with child subjects have been dealt with in the chapter by Jan Storch. Medical issues of improving prenatal and perinatal care and utilizing various forms of treatment are beyond the scope of this chapter. The primary nursing issues in caring for the small newborn infant have been identified as the promotion of physical and cognitive development, and the promotion of parent-infant attachment.

An overview will be given of the nature and scope of the problem of low birthweight infants in Canada. Promotion of physical and cognitive development will be examined in light of the current research on infant stimulation and the findings of our own study of physically handling infants in the neonatal intensive care unit will be described. The promotion of parent-infant attachment will be discussed with a focus on the effects of the separation of the infant and his parents and ways in which bonding can be enhanced in a highly specialized tertiary care unit. Finally, the implications of neonatal nursing in the future will be presented.

NATURE AND SCOPE OF THE PROBLEM

The World Health Organization clearly differentiates between infants who are preterm, i.e. born prior to the end of the 37th week of gestation, and those who are of low birthweight i.e. weighing less than 2500 g at birth. Since the majority of studies of neonatal course and outcome published prior to this time do not make a clear differentiation between these two factors, it is difficult to determine whether low birthweight, prematurity, or a combination of the two are the risk factors of concern. For purposes of this chapter, the focus will be on the infant whose birthweight is below 2500 g while the influence of gestational age will be noted where significant. In Canada, the percentage of low birthweight babies has declined significantly over the past 15 years, from 7.8% of live births in 1966 to 6.1% in 1979. A difference related to gender continues to exist, with 6.7% of female infants weighing less than 2500 g at birth while only 5.5% of male infants fall into this category. As might be expected, an inverse relationship exists between the number of weeks of gestation and the percentage of low birthweight infants. At 32–35 weeks gestation, 67% of infants weigh less than 2500 g, at 36–39 weeks only 8% are low birthweight, and at 40 weeks and beyond the figure is less than 2%.

The age of the mother appears related to the infant's birthweight with the highest percentage of low birthweight infants born to mothers less than 20 or greater than 40 years of age. Mothers between 25 and 34 years of age are at lowest risk for producing small babies, a statistic which has remained essentially unchanged for the last three decades in Canada (Statistics Canada, June 1982, p7).

The two major concerns in caring for the low birthweight infant are to keep the child alive, and to assist it in achieving an optimal level of health. Over the past 20 years in Canada (1959 to 1979) the number of infant deaths has been reduced by 70%. Deaths during the perinatal period have decreased by 69%, neonatal deaths are down by 70%, and deaths beyond the 28th day of life have been reduced by 72%. Earlier and better prenatal care, fetal monitoring, and close supervision during labour and delivery, as well as the advent of neonatal intensive care units are factors which have contributed to lowering the infant death rate.

Clearly then, the focus of health care workers should be on reducing the morbidity and increasing the quality of life for the low birthweight infant. Wille & Obladen (1981, p267) reviewed a large number of neonatal follow-up studies from around the world and came to the following conclusions: studies done in the 1950s showed 50% of preterm infants to have neurological impairment; by the 1960s this figure had fallen to 35%, and by the 1970s only 10–20% of infants were impaired. The authors are quick to point out the dangers in comparing studies based on a wide variation in study subjects, methods of care, definitions of impairment, and length of follow-up. The general trend toward a reduction in impairment, however, is probably a positive indication of improving outcome. A study of 101 preterm infants published in 1982 by Trotter et al found 18% of the infants to have mental or motor developmental delays at one year, a figure which supports the trend noted by Wille & Obladen.

INFANT STIMULATION

Infant stimulation has been suggested as one way to promote physical and cognitive development in the preterm or low birthweight infant. Research studies are described using various forms and combinations of visual, auditory, tactile, and vestibular stimulation. Outcome measures differ and length of follow-up varies, making results difficult to interpret.

Prior to 1970, only three studies appear in the literature which deal with the effects of handling or stimulation on infant human subjects. Hasselmeyer, in 1964, performed a classic study of the effects of increased tactile and kinesthetic stimulation of preterm infants. In this study, 60 preterm infants were randomly selected and assigned to either a control group which received routine nursery handling or to an experimental group which received extra rocking, cuddling, and stroking. Infants in the experimental group were found to be more quiescent, especially before feeding, while control infants exhibited more crying before feeds. There were no differences between the groups in morbidity, weight gain, number of defecations, or response to the interruption of a feeding. Hasselmeyer's study, which demonstrated positive effects of stimulation, challenged the prevalent belief in minimal handling.

Solkoff et al (1969) report on an unpublished study by Freedman, Boverman, and Freedman (1966) in which five sets of twins were given differential handling. One twin was rocked for 30 minutes twice a day for 7–10 days, and the second twin received routine nursery care. The rocked infant gained weight at a greater rate than his control in every group, although this trend did not persist beyond six months of age.

In 1969, Solkoff and his group studied ten low birthweight infants to determine the immediate and long-term effects of handling on behavioural and physical development. Experimental infants received five minutes of stroking every hour for a total of ten days while control infants received routine nursery care. Handled infants were more active, and cried less than the control infants. The handled infants also regained their birthweights faster although their initial advantage was lost by six weeks of age.

Both groups of babies were followed up at 7–8 months of age by medical staff who had no knowledge of the study. The handled children surpassed controls on both physical examination and the Bayley Test of Motor and Mental Development. Home studies also revealed that greater stimulation and mother-infant interaction occurred in the environments of the handled infants.

By the 1970s, the forms of stimulation being offered to infants had become more complex. Barnard (1973) studied 15 preterm infants with birthweights ranging from 1269–2453 g. The experimental group of 7 infants were stimulated by mechanical rocking in the isolette and a recorded heartbeat for 15 minutes each hour over a 14 day period. Experimental subjects showed a greater gain in quiet sleep and a larger reduction in the active awake state than the control subjects.

Neal (1977) provided various forms of vestibular stimulation to four groups of five preterm infants ranging in gestational age from 28–32 weeks. Group A infants were placed in a hammock which was swung for 30 minutes, three times a day; group B infants were placed in a hammock which they could swing themselves by moving; group C infants were placed in a stationary hammock, and group D infants were given routine care. The study continued until the infants were 36 weeks of age. Infants in group A had the highest scores for general maturation. In addition, these infants achieved and maintained a normal pH earlier than infants in other groups. Infants in group B showed the greatest increase in weight gain although this was not maintained throughout the first year of life.

The studies of stimulation described, and numerous others with different or additional forms of stimulation including music, tape recordings of mother's voice, stationary or rocking waterbeds, for example, share a common conceptual framework. The infant is seen as a passive individual upon whom is imposed active, one-sided stimulation. The transactional model, by contrast, holds that 'the developing organism is an active participant in its own progress, which it effects by imposing change upon its total environment and reacting to the new situation it has created by some form of learning, consolidation, or other behaviour' (Fox, 1981, p.125). The most important participants in this form of transactional stimulation with the infant are his parents. Unless parents are taught to recognize the unique needs of their infant and the cues that he gives regarding his readiness for and tolerance of stimulation, then it is likely that stimulation programs will be of little benefit.

The reasons for teaching stimulation to parents, however, should be very clear. There is no evidence that neurological damage can be undone by external influence or that repair of the nervous system can be enhanced by in-put. The greatest value of stimulation may, in fact, be the promotion of parent-infant attachment which leads to greater interaction and subsequent benefits for the child's development.

In low birthweight infants, the quality of parenting is believed to be the most important variable in predicting neurological outcome. Correlations between outcome and obstetrical factors or medical conditions hold true for the first two years of life but fade beyond that age in the presence of adequate parenting (Fox, 1981).

In planning a parent-infant stimulation program for the low birthweight infant, it is crucial to match the sensori-motor input to the receptive capacity of the child. The infant of 28 weeks gestation, for example, is challenged to maintain physiological homeostasis in the face of both internal and external stressors. The child responds to stimulation with alterations in physiological parameters which are readily observed and measured. By 34–36 weeks gestation, the infant begins to gain motor control and can respond to stimulation with patterned rather than random movements (Minde, 1978b). At this age, however, the infant may react aversively or protectively to stimuli which are appropriate to a more mature child (Fox, 1981).

The preterm infant at 44 weeks post-conceptional age is usually able to maintain, or to transfer between, various states of arousal. The quiet alert state is first seen at this age and the infant is ready for appropriate stimulation (Fox, 1981). It is important to note that the infant is now able to defend himself against noxius stimuli.

In addition to considering increased stimulation for this group of infants, however, environmentally imposed levels of stimulation must be considered. Sell (1980) describes the Neonatal Intensive Care environment as a relentless barrage of negative stimuli which includes constant ambient light and noise. Environmental noise caused by incubators, monitors, life support equipment, telephones, and staff activities has been shown to cause hypoxemia and increased intracranial pressure in infants in NICU (Long et al 1980). Handling, although necessary for the care of infants might also be considered a negative stimulus.

A number of investigators have demonstrated that handling resulting in movement, struggling or crying can lead to irregular respirations, tachycardia, and a marked fall in arterial oxygen in the compromised infant (Dangman et al, 1976; Speidel, 1978; Dinwiddie et al, 1979). Dangman et al (1976) and Speidel et al (1978) demonstrated that a series of procedures in close succession caused prolonged hypoxemia, which persisted for as long as seven minutes before arterial oxygen returned to baseline values.

THE EDMONTON STUDY

The Edmonton study was undertaken to determine the nature, duration, and frequency of handling of critically ill preterm infants in a neonatal intensive care unit. The effects of handling on the infant, as measured by changes in heart rate, mean arterial blood pressure, intracranial pressure, and arterial oxygen tension (PaO_2) were continuously recorded on a four channel recorder for a total of 24 hours for each study infant. A skeletal muscle relaxant (pancuronium bromide) was administered to the infants for 12 of the 24 hours to determine whether muscle relaxation would attenuate the effects of handling. Infants received the drug during the first or second 12 hour period based on random assignment. The study periods were separated by 12 hours to ensure that there were no lingering effects of the drug.

The study subjects constituted a population of 10 infants who had a gestational age of 37 weeks or less, a birthweight of 801–2000 g, and respiratory distress requiring mechanical ventilation and an inspired oxygen concentration of 40% or greater.

Throughout the study all nursing care given to the infants was observed and recorded using a continuous observation tool* designed specifically for use in a neonatal intensive care unit. The tool described nine major categories of nursing care including: hygiene, positioning, pulmonary care, special procedures, blood sampling, assistance with X-rays, medications, soothing, and a miscellaneous category for any additional procedures which did not appear on the list.

Reason for the study

The preterm, low birthweight infant is well known to be at risk for both immediate and long-term developmental problems. Many of these problems were discovered, upon further investigation, to be iatrogenic in nature, resulting from well-meaning but potentially harmful efforts to preserve the infant's life (Lucey et al, 1977). In addition, there is growing evidence that seemingly innocuous, routine procedures employed in the care of the preterm neonate can have a profound effect on the infant's condition. Changing a diaper, for example, has been shown to drop the infant's oxygen tension

*Available on request from author

($P0_2$) by as much as 30 torr (Peabody et al, 1978). Performing a number of procedures in close succession appears to have an additive effect in producing hypoxemia (Speidel, 1978). Hypoxemia in the preterm infant is believed to result mainly from the shunting of blood from the venous to the arterial side of the circulation. Shortly after birth this occurs through the foramen ovale and patent ductus arteriosus. Later, it more commonly occurs at the pulmonary level resulting from the perfusion of atelectatic areas of the lung (Speidel, 1978).

Decreased arterial oxygen has been demonstrated to increase pulmonary vascular resistance, reduce perfusion of the lung and keep the ductus arteriosus open. Heymann & Hoffman (1979) found that the greater the degree of hypoxia, the more rapid the rise in pulmonary vascular resistance.

In the preterm infant, the response to hypoxia remains paradoxical for about three weeks (Bryan & Bryan, 1979). When the preterm infant is challenged with hypoxia, ventilation increases within 30 seconds indicating that the peripheral chemoreceptors are intact. Ventilation then decreases within five minutes suggesting that the peripheral effect is later overruled by the central depressant effect of hypoxia. This biphasic response does not alter with gestational age but is influenced by postnatal age. By 18 days of age, preterm infants respond to hypoxia with sustained hyperventilation (Rigatto, 1979).

Movement struggling, and crying in response to handling also results in tachycardia, irregular respirations, and increased intracranial pressure (Long et al, 1980). Recent evidence suggests that fluctuations in arterial oxygen tension, blood pressure, and intracranial pressure may be associated with hypoxic brain damage and intracranial hemorrhage (Reynolds et al, 1979). If these theories are correct, then diminishing or eradicating the infant's motor response to handling should help to maintain his vital signs and level of oxygenation within a homeostatic range despite his need for physical care.

Care of the paralyzed infant

Pharmacologically induced skeletal muscle relaxation was considered as one possible way of reducing alterations in oxygenation and intracranial pressure when handling of the infant is necessary. Pancuronium bromide (Pavulon®) is a neuromuscular blocking agent which has been of value in the management of mechanically ventilated neonates. Use of the drug has been shown to improve ventilation and oxygenation and to lower the incidence of pneumothorax (Stark et al, 1979). Nursing care for the infant receiving pancuronium bromide is critical for that patient's survival. Should the ventilator fail to function for any reason or inadvertently become disconnected from the infant's airway, the child will be unable to breathe on his own. The nurse must be frequently and particularly observant of the condition of the patient, the respiratory rate, and the ventilator settings. Alarms on the ventilator should always be turned on and the nurse should have a clear understanding of what they mean. A resuscitation bag, mask, and oxygen must be at the bedside at all times in case of emergency.

The infant may need suctioning more frequently than usual since pancuronium bromide increases both pharyngeal and tracheal secretions. Instillation of half strength normal saline prior to suctioning may facilitate the procedure by reducing the tenacity of secretions, although the risks resulting from airway obstruction are of concern in the compromised infant. Effective hydration is essential and in some instances chest physiotherapy and postural drainage are of benefit.

Attention must be paid to the infant's patterns of elimination. Although pancuronium bromide does not affect the smooth muscle of the urinary bladder, periodic manual expression of urine does appear to be necessary for the newborn. The muscles of the anal sphincter are paralyzed by the drug, however, and the nurse will need to assist with bowel evacuation if the infant is being fed.

Skin breakdown can occur rapidly due to the fragility of the small preterm infant's skin, and his inability to move. This may be further aggravated if peripheral perfusion is poor. Infants should be repositioned at least every hour to change the weight bearing areas of his body. The blink reflex is absent when an infant is receiving pancuronium as its use leads to drying of the cornea. Artificial tears and the application of eye patches help to maintain corneal integrity and minimize the potential risk of eye damage.

Although the infant has no control over motor function, his sensory perception remains intact and his level of consciousness is not altered by pancuronium. This should be kept in mind when the nurse is performing procedures which may be distressing or painful to the infant. Occasionally sedation is ordered in conjunction with pancuronium (Kravitz & Pace, 1979). Parents who may already be upset about the infant's condition may need reassurance that it is still important to touch and talk to their child. They may become dis-

couraged by the lack of response to their handling, and visit the
NICU less often. The nurse can play a crucial role in maintaining
and promoting parent-infant attachment in these circumstances.

Findings of the study

Description of nursing care

The data on the frequency and duration of handling were consistent
with the findings of previous studies. The mean number of contacts
per infant was 105 in 24 hours, a figure slightly lower than the 132
contacts in 24 hours described by Korones (1976). The mean duration of contact per baby, however, was higher in the present study
being 265 minutes per baby per 24 hours compared to 238 minutes
per baby in Korones' study. It appears that technological advances
in critical care such as continuous monitoring of vital signs and PO_2
have done little to diminish the frequency and duration of disturbance for the infant. Future development of monitoring techniques
for CO_2 and pH may further disrupt the infant's periods of rest.

Nursing care was categorized and ranked according to frequency
of occurrence (Table 6.1). Airway suctioning was the most time
consuming procedure with each infant being suctioned for an average of 60 minutes in 24 hours. This accounted for 23% of the nursing
care the infant received. In light of the close relationship between
suctioning and hypoxia, nurses should consider ways in which the
procedure could be modified to maintain a more stable PO_2. In the
NICU where the study was conducted, it was common practice to
increase the inspired oxygen for 1–2 minutes prior to suction. Despite the resulting rise in PO_2, however, suctioning produced prolonged periods of hypoxia followed by rebounds of hyperoxia.

The handling of equipment, including such nursing activities as
applying chest leads, inserting an intravenous catheter, and calibrat-
ing a blood pressure transducer ranked closely behind suctioning in
causing disturbance to the infants and accounting for 20% of total
care. Such concentration on the mechanical aspects of care may
contribute to altered parent-infant attachment as described in a
subsequent section.

Approximately 13% of the infants' care consisted of obtaining
blood samples. Arterial blood gas samples, drawn from the umbilical
artery catheter were the most frequent samples required. While this
may appear to be an inordinate percentage of total care, it involves
only 32 minutes in a 24 hour period. Considering the acuity of illness

Table 6.1 Categories of handling ranked according to duration and percentage of time spent on each

Pancuronium

Handling	Time spent (minutes)	Percentage of total time
Suctioning	312	24.06
Handling equipment	247	19.04
Vital signs	175	13.49
Blood sampling	172	13.26
Hygiene	91	7.02
Medications	78	6.01
Physical exam	63	4.86
Soothing	59	4.55
Weighing	42	3.24
Diagnostic procedures	34	2.62
Physiotherapy	24	1.85
All handling	1297	100.00

Control

Handling	Time spent (minutes)	Percentage of total time
Suctioning	293	21.66
Handling equipment	289	21.36
Blood sampling	187	13.82
Vital signs	173	12.79
Soothing	100	7.39
Hygiene	95	7.02
Physical exam	74	5.47
Weighing	54	3.99
Medications	45	3.33
Diagnostic procedures	37	2.73
Physiotherapy	6	0.44
All handling	1353	100.00

of the infants studied and the dangers of both high and low arterial oxygen levels, the procedure does not seem inappropriate although marked increases in intracranial pressure resulting from flushing of the arterial line were cause for concern. Heelstick samples for blood sugar, although causing a marked change in the infants' physiologic parameters, usually occurred only once per shift. A further 13% of care involved checking vital signs. Again, this seems appropriate for critically ill babies even though they are monitored continuously. Other aspects of care took a much smaller percentage of the nurses' time and are illustrated in Table 6.1.

Relationship of nursing care to altered physiologic parameters

Changes in heart rate, mean arterial blood pressure, arterial oxygen, and intracranial pressure were considered in relation to whether the changes occurred when the infant was receiving pancuronium or during the control period when he was free to respond to stimulation. Heart rate and blood pressure were not found to differ between the two periods, but statistically significant relationships were seen between the other physiologic parameters, and specific types of nursing care (Table 6.2).

Table 6.2 Nursing procedures which were significantly related to changes in physiologic parameters

Physiologic change (duration)	Nursing procedure (duration)	Pancuronium (P) or Control (C)	Pearsons r	t value	Significance
Hypoxia	Diagnostic procedures	P	.77	3.44	P<.001
	Suctioning	C	.71	2.84	p<.02
	Weighing	C	.60	2.12	p<.05
Hyperoxia	Weighing	P	.63	2.30	p<.02
	Hygiene	C	.64	2.36	p<.02
	TLC	C	.55	1.86	p<.05
Increased intracranial pressure	Vital signs	P	.62	2.23	p<.05
	TLC	P	.69	2.68	p<.02

Hypoxia, defined as a PO_2 less than 50 torr, resulted from diagnostic procedures when the infants were on pancuronium and from suctioning and weighing during the control period. The diagnostic procedures were primarily chest X-rays. These tended to be prolonged procedures lasting about 10 minutes and involving a great deal of handling of the infant and several changes in position. During such times endotracheal tubes frequently became kinked or disconnected from the ventilator when babies were paralyzed and unable to breathe spontaneously. Close observation of the position and connections of airway control tubing are essential for preventing hypoventilation leading to hypoxia.

Two of the infants studied had a marked fall in core temperature during the procedures, probably resulting from the movement of the overhead radiant heat source away from the bed to facilitate placement of the X-ray machine. Placing the infants on cool X-ray plates may also have contributed to conductive heat loss. Checking the infant's rectal and skin temperatures immediately following an X-ray, and ensuring that X-ray plates are wrapped in bubble plastic or a diaper are advisable precautions in averting cold stress. Cold stress increases oxygen uptake and further compromises the hypoxic infant.

Suctioning causes hypoxia by removing oxygen and by obstructing the airway. Frequent or prolonged suctioning leads to profound hypoxia, and it may take as long as 12 minutes for oxygen levels to return to baseline values. It is surprising that hypoxia during suction was so greatly reduced when the infants were paralyzed, particularly in light of their increased secretions. This finding suggests that struggling and crying play an even greater role in hypoxia than previously believed. Bradycardia resulting from suctioning is also of concern since the newborn is unable to increase his stroke volume. Decreased heart rate therefore results in decreased cardiac output, further contributing to hypoxia.

The relationship between hypoxia and weighing may be less obvious. In the course of this procedure infants are removed from the ventilator to be placed on a scale at the bedside. The decision as to whether the infant receives oxygen or manual ventilation at this time is left to the discretion of the nurse. An infant on pancuronium is unable to breathe spontaneously and the nurse is therefore more likely to bag the paralyzed infant. It is during the control period when no assistance is given that the baby becomes hypoxic. Observing the PO_2 monitor closely during weighing and maintaining a stable level of oxygenation is an important nursing responsibility. An infant who requires oxygen and assisted ventilation should never be removed from the ventilator for procedures such as X-rays or weighing.

Hyperoxia has been associated with both lung and eye damage in the newborn. While the level and duration of hyperoxia which results in complications is not known, it is believed that maintaining the PO_2 below 70 torr is desirable. In the present study, hyperoxia was associated with weighing when the babies were on pancuronium bromide and with hygiene and soothing during the control period. The relationship with weighing seems to be a side effect of nursing care previously described: removal from the ventilator, and indiscriminate bagging. Manual ventilation and/or the administration of oxygen to the paralyzed infant, when not coupled with close monitoring of PO_2 can result in excessive oxygenation.

The observed relationships between hyperoxia and hygiene or soothing is more difficult to interpret. If these types of nursing care are viewed as comfort measures, then it may be that the infant's level of arousal is lowered and he may stop crying or fall asleep. Vidyasagar & Asonye (1979) suggest this would in turn decrease shunting and raise the infant's PO_2 even with the same inspired oxygen concentration.

Increased intracranial pressure, defined as a level of 10 or more cm H_2O above baseline, was related to taking vital signs and soothing the infants when they were receiving pancuronium. The association with vital signs is postulated to result from the nurse holding the infant's feet in the air to insert a rectal thermometer. Raising the feet causes increased cerebral blood flow thereby increasing intracranial pressure. It is further suggested that the relationship does not hold true during the control period because the normal muscle tone of the diaphragm minimizes the pressure of the abdominal contents on the thoracic organs, maintaining normal blood flow and intracranial pressure.

The relationship between raised intracranial pressure and soothing appears less logical. On two occasions an abrupt rise in pressure was noted when infants first heard their mother's voice or had physical contact with her. We may have been observing a physiologic response to pleasurable sensation, exaggerated in the paralyzed infant because he has no other outlet for expression.

Conclusions

No differences were found in the frequency and duration of handling during administration of pancuronium and control periods. During both study periods infants did experience periods of hypoxia, hyperoxia, and increased intracranial pressure in response to handling. The degree of fluctuation beyond physiological bounds is significantly reduced by the administration of a skeletal muscle relaxant, and may lead to a decrease in sequelae in the high risk infant.

PROMOTION OF PARENT-INFANT ATTACHMENT

To this point, discussion has focused on the interaction of the low birthweight infant with professional staff. The effects of both planned stimulation and handling associated with nursing care have been described. It is crucial, however, for staff to assist and support the parents in their role as primary caregivers for the infant.

Fox (1981) defined parenting as 'the ability of mothers and fathers to understand, anticipate, and make mutually satisfactory adaptations to the individual personality and needs of their offspring so as to enhance achievement of developmental goals' (p.136). It is suggested that the parents of a preterm or low birthweight infant may have more difficulty in understanding, anticipating, and adapting to their infant's needs than the parents of a healthy fullterm newborn, and that this may lead to parenting difficulties. Kennell & Klaus (1980) report that 25–41% of children who fail to thrive and 23–31% of battered children were born prematurely.

Dr Klaus Minde, a child psychiatrist, refutes two of the major studies on which such findings were based. He states that Elmer & Gregg (1967) gave only a vague definition of abuse and that they experienced a substantial loss of study subjects in that 30 of the 50 children in their study were lost to follow-up. In response to Klein & Stern's classic study (1971) linking abuse and prematurity, Minde points out that 50% of the study subjects had associated chronic medical problems or mental retardation which might more appropriately have been precipitating factors for abuse.

Studies linking prematurity with failure to thrive were criticized by Minde for having included among subjects, infants whose height and/or weight were already below the 3rd percentile for their age. The investigators also failed to differentiate between infants who were appropriate and those who were small for their gestational age at birth. In the studies reviewed, none of the children showed a change in their growth patterns. While the link between low birthweight and later abuse and neglect may be tenuous, however, it is beneficial to consider the factors influencing parent-infant attachment in this group.

Parental reaction to preterm birth

Premature delivery has been described by Caplan et al (1977) as a crisis situation which creates feelings of depression and guilt in parents. A study by Harper et al (1974) of parents whose infants were cared for in NICU further describes parental reactions of denial, rejection, and fear. Expression of such feelings is normal, and is prognostic of good psychosocial adjustment to the birth of an at-risk infant (Caplan et al, 1977).

Four psychological tasks which the mother must complete if she is to establish a healthy relationship with her sick newborn have been described by Kaplan & Mason (1977). These tasks are: preparation for the possible loss of the child, acknowledgement of her failure to deliver a healthy, fullterm infant, resumption of the process of relating to the child, and understanding the special needs and growth patterns of the preterm infant. It is believed that the first two tasks must be completed before the mother can bond effectively with her infant.

Psychological preparation for loss has been termed anticipatory grief and has been shown to be pervasive among parents of infants in NICU, even when the infant's life is not in jeopardy (Benfield et al 1976). Klaus & Kennell (1982) feel that parental grief reactions are eased, and bonding to the infant promoted, by early contact and frequent visits to the NICU. Recent work by Taylor & Hall (1979) suggests, however, that the grief response occurs irrespective of separation and that it is still present when mothers deliver in a tertiary centre and have unrestricted access to their infants.

Helping parents to deal with their feelings of grief and failure can be done through individual counselling or through group meetings with other parents. Minde and his group (1978a) found a weekly self-help group for parents helped to attenuate the psychological pain associated with the crisis of having a premature infant. Weekly group meetings were coordinated by an experienced neonatal nurse and attended by a 'veteran mother' who had had a small infant in NICU during the previous 12–15 months. The groups met for 7–12 weeks. Mothers who attended the group visited the nursery significantly more often, interacted more with their infants during visits, and felt more competent about their general caretaking role than control mothers.

There is evidence that the number of visits mothers make to their infants in NICU is predictive of later maternal interactive behaviours (Minde, 1978a), but it must also be recognized that being in the intensive care environment can be very stressful for parents.

Dr Rita Harper and her colleagues (1974) administered a 63 item questionnaire to the parents of 100 infants cared for in the intensive care nursery. The responses to the questionnaire indicated a good deal of anxiety related to visiting a child in the intensive care nursery and that anxiety increased in direct proportion to the number of visits. The degree of parental stress related directly to the severity of illness and the prognosis for the infant. Stress was found to relate also to the nursery environment, the perceived support of nursery personnel, and the extent of parent-infant contact. Despite the anxiety, however, most parents were strongly in favour of open visiting policies.

Mothers who are not able to visit infants have been shown to demonstrate difficulties in the areas of commitment to the infant, self-confidence in the ability to mother the infant, and behaviour toward the infant such as stimulation and interaction (Barnett et al, 1970). Such findings have raised concerns regarding the separation of mother and infant shortly after birth.

Separation and the 'sensitive period'

A number of authors have attested to the value of maternal-infant contact during the first few hours following birth. Based on animal studies, Klaus & Kennell (1970) have suggested the existence of a sensitive period following birth during which attachment is initiated, although in their later writings (1982) they have modified their earlier position that this period is critical to bonding. Based on this tenet, however, clinicians who deal with families of low birthweight infants have become concerned with the separation of parents and infants which is necessitated by the treatment of the child in a highly specialized centre and have sought ways of facilitating both early and continuing contact between parents and infants.

The benefits of early and extended contact include prolonged breast feeding and increased affectionate behaviours such as face-to-face looking, kissing, and fondling. Infants who experience increased contact cry less, smile more, and perform better on standard developmental tests. In one study of 301 low income primiparous mothers there was a suggestion that greater contact prevented the subsequent occurrence of child abuse (Ross, 1980).

Ross suggests, however, that the body of research upon which these conclusions are based has some serious methodological and theoretical difficulties. Sample sizes are small and positive outcomes have not been found to persist. Dependent variables differ and have not all been validated as measures of successful attachment. Further, the appropriateness of applying an animal model to human behaviour has been questioned. Richards (1978) and Rutter (1979) argue that the mother's perception of and attitudes toward separation are more important determinants of behaviour than the separation itself.

Behaviour of the low birthweight infant

Reducing the degree of separation between parents and infant and encouraging visits to the NICU are two methods of promoting attachment and assisting parents to resume their relationship with their infant. It is essential, however, that parents know the kind of behaviour they might expect from the preterm, low birthweight infant. The premature infant, at term, is more hypotonic or hyperactive than normal fullterm infants; he is more difficult to arouse, and once aroused, to soothe; he is less apt to orient to a face or a voice; and his grasping and sucking responses are weaker (Ross, 1980).

Unless parents clearly understand what to expect from their infants, they may be disappointed or shocked by newborn behaviour and may not form an effective attachment. Minde and his group (1980) have further emphasized that infants are largely non-responsive to social interactions prior to 34 weeks gestational age. Parents should be helped to understand that immature babies are unable, not unwilling, to respond to parental overtures.

Parents feel important to small infants when they are able to carry out normally expected behaviours such as feeding, bathing, and diapering. Mothers may feel incompetent or at very least, uncomfortable performing these tasks in the environment of the intensive care nursery where proficient and confident nursing staff may assume these roles. Nursing staff may sometimes be insensitive to the needs and skills of the mother to care for her own infant and may in fact promote the appearance of competent professionalism to the detriment of the mother-infant relationship. Parents must be encouraged to actively participate in the care of their infants and to share in decision making, and staff must assist and support the parents rather than creating an impression of being expert, authoritarian, or essential. If not dealt with, the mother's feelings of isolation and lack of control over the care of her own infant may extend beyond discharge.

The use of the Brazelton Neonatal Assessment Scale in the presence of the parents has been shown by Widmayer & Field (1981) to facilitate early interaction between parents and the newborn which may ultimately promote cognitive development of the infant. The investigators studied 30 healthy preterm infants who were randomly assigned to one of three groups. One group invited parents to be present during a Brazelton Assessment of their child and complete the Mother's Assessment of the Behaviour of her Infant Scale (MABI) at birth and weekly for 4 weeks following discharge. The second experimental group completed the MABI but were not present during the Brazelton Assessment, and the control group parents were asked to complete a questionnaire on the developmental milestones of their infants.

Home visits were carried out at 1, 4, and 12 months, and significant differences in interaction were observed. At 1 month, the experimental infants excelled on the Brazelton Scale and were rated more highly on videotaped sequences of feeding and face-to-face play. The experimental infants showed better fine motor adaptive abilities on the Denver Development Screening Test (DDST) at 4 months and scored higher on the Bayley Scales of mental development at 12 months. The authors concluded that demonstrating the abilities of the preterm infant to the parents can be of benefit. While learning the techniques necessary to the appropriate administration of assessment tools is time consuming and requires considerable skill, it is well within the scope of nursing practice to learn and to utilize such skills to assist parents in bonding with their high risk infant.

SUMMARY

The outlook for the low birthweight infant is improving, as evidenced by steadily declining rates of mortality and morbidity. Since obstetrical and neonatal factors are predictive of outcome only for the first 2 years of life, however, there must be a number of other factors which influence the child's physical and cognitive development.

Planned infant stimulation programs using a variety of sensory modalities have been associated with accelerating some aspects of development, although long-term follow-up studies are needed to determine whether the effects persist. Caution must be exercised in developing stimulation programs to ensure that they are appropriate to the infant's stage of neurological development. Involving parents in the program may encourage continued interaction with the infant after discharge.

Attachment of parents to their low birthweight infant is influenced by the crisis of premature delivery, separation from the infant during the first hours after birth, and the infant's limited behavioural repetorie. Nurses may help to promote bonding by encouraging visiting in the NICU and involving the parents in the care of their child. Demonstrating newborn abilities for the parents and explaining behaviour as resulting from immaturity rather than abnormality has been shown to improve parents' confidence in caring for their newborn. Parent support groups have also been beneficial in promoting attachment.

Much more work needs to be done in the areas of parent education and planning for discharge. Most of the literature to date is anecdotal but does describe the parents' need for assistance, support, and early follow-up at this crucial time. A great deal of progress has been made in perinatal and neonatal medicine to improve the lot of the low birthweight infant. The role of nursing has just begun.

REFERENCES

Barnard K 1973 The effect of stimulation on the sleep behaviour of the premature infant. In: Batey M (ed) Communicating nursing research: Collaboration and competition. Western Interstate Commission for Higher Education, Boulder, Colorado

Barnett C R, Liederman P H, Grobstein R, Klaus M 1970 Neonatal separation: The maternal side of interactional deprivation. Pediatrics 45: 197–204

Benfield D G, Lieb S A, Reuter J 1976 Grief response of parents after referral of the critically ill newborn to a regional centre. New England Journal of Medicine 294: 975–978

Bryan A C, Bryan M H 1979 Control of respiration in the newborn. In: Thibeault D W, Gregory G A (eds) Neonatal pulmonary care. Addison Wesley, Don Mills, Ontario

Caplan G, Mason E A, Kaplan D M 1977 Four studies of crisis in parents of prematures. In: Schwartz J H, Schwartz L H (eds) Vulnerable infants. A psychosocial dilemma. McGraw-Hill, New York, p 89–107

Dangman B C, Hegyi T, Hyatt M 1976 The variability of P0$_2$ in newborn infants in response to routine care (abstract). Pediatric Research 10: 422

Dinwiddie R, Patel B D, Kumar S P, Fox W W 1979 The effects of crying on arterial oxygen tension in infants recovering from respiratory distress. Critical Care Medicine 7: 50–53

Elmer E, Gregg G S 1967 Developmental characteristics of abused children. Pediatrics 40: 596–602

Fox M 1981 Assessment for sensori-motor stimulation. In: Proceedings of the third symposium on the prevention of handicapping conditions of prenatal and perinatal origin. Alberta Social Services and Community Health, Edmonton

Harper R G, Concepcion S, Sokal S, Sokal M 1974 Observations on unrestricted parental contact with infants in the neonatal intensive care unit. Journal of Pediatrics 3: 441–445

Hasselmeyer E G 1964 Handling and premature infant behaviour (Doctoral dissertation New York University, 1963). Ann Arbor: Xerox

Heymann M A, Hoffman J E 1979 Pulmonary circulation in the perinatal period. In: Thibeault D W, Gregory G A (eds) Neonatal pulmonary care. Addison-Wesley, Don Mills, Ontario

Kaplan D M, Mason E A 1977 Maternal reactions to premature birth viewed as an acute emotional disorder. In: Schwartz J H, Schwartz L H (eds) Vulnerable infants. A psychosocial dilemma. McGraw-Hill, New York, p 80–88

Kennell J, Klaus M 1980 Parenting in the premature nursery. In: Sell E J (ed) Follow-up of the high risk newborn. A practical approach. Thomas, Springfield, p 180–186

Klaus M, Kennell J 1970 Mothers separated from their newborn infants. Pediatric Clinics of North America 17: 1015–1037

Klaus M, Kennell J 1982 Parent-infant bonding, 2nd edn. Mosby, St Louis

Klein M, Stern L 1971 Low birth weight and the battered child syndrome. American Journal of Diseases in Children 122: 15–18

Korones S B 1976 Disturbances and infants' rest. In: Moore T C (ed) Iatrogenic problems in neonatal intensive care. Report of the sixty-ninth Ross Conference on Pediatric Research. Ross Laboratories, Columbus, Ohio

Kravitz M, Pace N L 1979 Management of the mechanically ventilated patient receiving pancuronium bromide. Heart and Lung 8: 81–86

Long J G, Lucey J F, Philip A G S 1980 Noise and hypoxemia in the intensive care nursery. Pediatrics 65: 143–145

Lucey J T, Peabody J L, Philip A G S 1977 Recurrent undetected hypoxia and hyperoxia: A newly recognized iatrogenic problem of 'intensive care'. (abstract). Pediatric Research 11: 537

Minde K 1980 Bonding of mothers to premature infants: Theory and practice. In: Taylor P M (ed) Parent infant relationships. Grune & Stratton, New York, p 291–314

Minde K, Shosenberg N, Marton P, Hines B, Shanoff J 1978a Self-help groups in a premature nursery — A controlled evaluation paper presented at the annual meeting of the American Orthopsychiatric Association, San Francisco

Minde K, Trehub S, Corter C, Boukydis C, Celhoffer L, Marton P 1978b Mother-child relationships in a premature nursery: An observational study. Pediatrics 61: 373–379

Neal M V 1977 Vestibular stimulation and development of the small premature infant. In: Batey M (ed) Communicating nursing research: Nursing research priorities: Choice or chance. Western Interstate Commission for Higher Education, Boulder, Colorado

Peabody J L, Willis M M, Gregory G A 1978 Clinical limitations and advantages of transcutaneous oxygen electrodes. Acta Anaesthesia Scandinavica (Suppl) 76–82

Reynolds M L, Evans C A N, Reynolds E O R 1979 Intracranial hemorrhage in the preterm sheep fetus. Early Human Development 3: 163–186

Richards M P M 1978 Possible effects of early separation on later development of children — a review. Clinics in Developmental Medicine 68: 12–32

Rigatto H 1979 Apnea. In: Thibeault D W, Gregory G A (eds) Neonatal pulmonary care. Addison-Wesley, Don Mills, Ontario, p 361–371

Ross G S 1980 Parental responses to infants in intensive care: The separation issue reevaluated. Clinics in Perinatology 7: 47–60

Rutter M 1979 Separation experiences. A new look at an old topic. Journal of Pediatrics 95: 147–154

Sell E J (ed) 1980 Follow-up of the high risk newborn. A practical approach. Thomas, Springfield

Solkoff N, Yaffe S, Weintraub D 1969 Effects of handling on the subsequent development of premature infants. Developmental Psychology 1: 765–768

Speidel B D 1978 Adverse effects of routine procedures on preterm infants. The Lancet 8069: 864–866

Stark A R, Bascom R, Frantz I D 1979 Muscle relaxation in mechanically ventilated infants. Journal of Pediatrics 94: 439–443

Statistics Canada 1982 Catalogue 84–001. Quarterly 29: 6–7

Stewart A L, Reynolds E O R 1974 Improved prognosis for infants of very low birthweight. Pediatrics 54: 724–735

Taylor P M, Hall B L 1979 Parent-infant bonding: Problems and opportunities in a perinatal centre. Seminars in Perinatology 3: 73–84

Trotter C W, Chang P, Thompson T 1982 Perinatal factors and the developmental outcome of preterm infants. Journal of Obstetric, Gynecologic and Neonatal Nursing 11: 83–90

Vidyasagar D, Asonye U 1979 Critical care problems of the newborn. Practical aspects of transcutaneous oxygen monitoring. Critical Care Medicine 7: 149–152

Widmayer S M, Field T M 1981 Effects of Brazelton demonstrations for mothers on the development of preterm infants. Pediatrics 67: 711–714

Wille L, Obladen M 1981 Neonatal intensive care principles and guidelines. Springer-Verlag, Berlin

Parental attitudes to premature very low birthweight babies

INTRODUCTION

The birth of a premature baby often precipitates a family crisis, for which parents are quite unprepared. Parents increasingly expect pregnancy to be uneventful until the normal birth occurs at about the expected time of 40 weeks; their mental picture is likely to be of a perfect, idealized baby (Klaus & Fanaroff, 1979). In the eyes of most parents, the premature baby falls far short of their expectations and they may be expected to grieve for the loss of their perfect baby. (Kaplan & Mason, 1960). Many other expectations related to the entire birth experience are unfulfilled; feelings of anger, depression and guilt may continue long after all medical concern for the infant has disappeared. With the increased control over fertility that most couples now have, the premature birth may upset plans for birth at convenient time. Disruption of family function frequently encompasses any other children, grandparents, relatives and close friends.

The changing prognosis of premature infants and alteration in attitude to parents are most vividly exemplified by very low birthweight (VLBW) infants, those of birthweight under 1500 g. The potential for survival of such infants has almost doubled in the past 15 years (Kitchen et al, 1980). Initially, the prime concern was with technological advances that permitted not only survival but also reduced the prevalence of long-term iatrogenic sequelae.

The importance of parents in relation to the newborn infant was established long ago by Budin (1907); once personnel in neonatal intensive care units (NICU) had achieved some mastery of the techniques used in modern neonatal intensive care, the essential role of the parents was rediscovered and increasingly emphasised. Motivation for better care for parents had both altruistic and practical aspects; the former embraced a compassionate wish to minimize the emotional distress of the parents of premature babies; the latter aspect recognized that a premature infant after leaving hospital is exquisitely sensitive to an unfavourable environment and that accepting, loving, informed parents may be the baby's best insurance against such unfavourable influences.

Many authors have emphasised the importance of intervention in the intensive care unit and have outlined possible strategies for caring for parents (Mangurten et al, 1979; Yu et al, 1981; Klaus & Kennell, 1982). Indication of the effect of any new strategies requires that the views of consumers — in this case the parents — should be sought. The present study, a descriptive one, surveys a non-random sample of parents of very low birthweight infants. The aims of the study were to obtain parents' views on the services offered to them by the NICU personnel and to offer them the opportunity to suggest improvements.

One can assume that both neonatal intensive care units and parents have some underlying similarities that transcend national boundaries. Further, that parents are likely to react in similar ways whenever sophisticated neonatal care facilities are encountered. Therefore, the findings of this study may be of some use to all nurses who work with parents of very low birthweight infants.

STUDY METHOD

Material and need

The survey was conducted in a major maternity hospital of 350 midwifery beds. The number of births during the year in which the survey took place was 6097. 156 births were infants whose birthweighht was less than 1500 g and who survived the neonatal period. Because the NICU and Newborn Emergency Transport Service (NETS) facilities form part of this hospital's service, many patients who have received their antenatal care outside the hospital but who have special obstetric problems or threatened premature delivery, are referred to the hospital at or near the time of delivery.

The NICU has ten cots and the special nursery floor has an average daily occupancy of 52 babies. Visiting policy encourages parents to visit anytime throughout the 24 hours. Grandparents and siblings are admitted to the nursery one at a time accompanied by one parent.

Procedures

The permission of parents to be included in the survey was obtained, and no-one refused to be interviewed. Two semi-structured interviews were conducted by a nurse/midwife. The first took place on the nursery floor approximately 10 weeks after the birth, at which time the majority of babies were managing without life supports and were in a normal cot. The second interview was timed to give the mother at least 6 weeks at home with her baby and on this occasion mothers were seen in the hospital outpatient area.

The first interview obtained data in the following areas:

a. Demographic descriptive
b. Child-birth education and premature labour
c. Reactions, feelings and concerns in respect of the VLBW infant
d. Interactions with staff
e. Perception of facilities provided and of parents' unmet needs.

The second interview covered such areas as:

a. Preparation for taking baby home
b. Problems on homecoming
c. Accessibility of help
d. Parents' suggestions for improvement in services.

The interviews took approximately 1½ hours each.

The sample

The sample survey entered NICU between July and December 1979 and consisted of mothers of infants whose birthweight was less than 1500 g who were available for interview on one particular day of the week.

This sampling method was dictated by financial and time constraints which made representative sampling impossible. Altogether 33 families were included in the study. In each case it was the mother on whom the interview was focused, although during nine of the interviews fathers were present for the entire time; a total of 16 were able to contribute their viewpoint.

The main characteristics of the sample are described in Table 7.1. The maternal age ranged from 18–35 years, the mean age being 27.6. The occupations of the fathers ranged across the Congalton scale (1969) from 1–7 but the majority were tradesmen and skilled and unskilled workers. 17 of the families lived within the Melbourne metropolitan region and 16 were from country areas. 15 of the mothers had been booked for delivery at the hospital and 17 were transferred from outside practices. Only one mother was delivered elsewhere; her baby was transferred to the hospital because of her need for intensive care. 16 of the infants were the first liveborn baby in their family. The weight range of the group was from 620–1390 g.

Table 7.1 Social characteristics of families

Social characteristic	No.
Age of mothers	
range 18–35	
20	3
21–25	9
26–30	7
31–35	14
Social status of fathers*	
1	1
2	2
3	5
4	6
5	8
6	7
7	4
Patient status	
Delivered at hospital	32
Non-booked	17
Booked	15
Delivered elsewhere	1
Place of residence	
Metropolitan area	17
Country	16

*Congalton Classification (Congalton 1969)

Results

Antenatal education and preparation for premature labour

Because of the premature birth these mothers missed the opportunity for normal antenatal education. For the ten primagravidae this was unfortunate for they came to labour completely unprepared; it was not surprising that they were confused and frightened, as shown by one patient's comment: 'I had no idea what was happening, water had been coming out for two weeks. My doctor said to carry on normally.' She had no idea what to expect.

Only those who had previously experienced premature birth had some idea of what might be expected but it was still a frightening experience for those mothers. One commented, 'Our last boy was 30 weeks, so we knew what was going to happen, but only 27 weeks this time, was a real worry.'

Premature labour — understanding of process and management

In this area questions were designed to discover the level of the mother's understanding of her situation and its management, as well as her perception of the adequacy of information provided. The unexpected events experienced by these mothers were antepartum haemorrhage, rupture of membranes, abdominal pains and pre-eclampsia. 12 mothers felt their condition was adequately explained to them. Three were too ill to comprehend the information given and the remaining 18 said they were given information that they mis-understood or failed to comprehend. Illustrative of this last group are the following comments:

> I felt completely abandoned by the doctor I had booked (called himself a specialist). When the water broke he sent me here without a letter of introduction or explanation and without any explanation to me. I thought I was dying with a miscarriage, I was too frightened to ask. The doctor who put in the 'drip' told me it would stop it, so when the baby came I was really shocked.

and

> My doctor told me he had a 50/50 chance, he said he thought the baby was a good size for 30 weeks but that meant nothing to me. He also said that he would have to terminate the pregnancy because of my blood pressure. I thought 'termination' meant 'abortion', so I was very muddled.

Salbutamol

We were interested in how the mothers perceived salbutamol (Ventolin) which was given to 12 of them to slow down contractions. Eight complained of side effects of rapid heart beat. If this possibility had been explained they did not understand the explanation. One said, 'The effect of the salbutamol had not worn off during labour and I felt faint, "my whole body was palpitating".' Others felt unpleasant side effects could be tolerated if time was gained for the baby. 'I had "the shakes" for ages but it had gained him nearly 2 weeks, so it was worth it.'

Epidural anaesthesia

Epidural anaesthesia was used in 11 cases to give more obstetric control over the delivery. Again side effects were a problem. 'The labour pain was as bad as any labour before the epidural. That was okay until it started to wear off after the baby came; I had groin cramps and twitches in both legs all night.' And 'The epidural helped but I didn't like the "wearing off", pins and needles and jumpy legs.' Mothers felt that some of the side effects of both salbutamol and epidurals would have been more acceptable if they had been warned beforehand; in spite of the unpleasant side effects, most stated they would go through it again if it was to help the baby. Generally the labour experience of these mothers was not good, and, for those who were uninformed or misunderstood information, it was extremely unpleasant.

Pain

Mothers were asked to comment on their experience of pain in labour. Only four had very little pain and for 15 labour was painful or very painful. Five mothers had a caesarean birth and four of the five did not regret this.

Support in labour

14 mothers had their partner present at the birth and all found this a source of comfort, especially if the father was able to tell them their baby's sex.

Contact with baby in delivery room

21 mothers saw the baby but only four of those held the baby for a few seconds and six touched toes or fingers in the transport incubator (Portacot). 12, including the five Caesarean births, had no contact with the baby in the delivery room and they were regretful about this, although mostly they did not have to wait long for information from the paediatrician who had been in attendance.

The first visit to NICU to see the baby and feelings toward him

Many questions asked in this area were answered at length, followed by discussion, as it was considered important to give the mothers time to express themselves fully.

The timing. The timing of the first visit was satisfactory to 27 mothers, 25 of whom visited within 18 hours of the delivery, including two of the five who had had a Caesarean birth. Four women stated that in the opinion of the staff, they were not well enough to visit the NICU; they did not agree with this opinion, and all said they had felt well enough (including the three other women who had Caesarean births) to be taken to the nursery. Three were excessively fearful of visiting the NICU and waited until either the father of the baby or a close relative could accompany them. Only one woman who was delivered at a country hospital waited until 7 days after the birth to visit — this was following her own discharge from hospital. The lingering effect of epidural anaethesia was one of the main reasons for her not visiting the baby earlier.

First impressions. On their first visit the majority looked only at their own baby, not noticing other babies, the bustle of the nursery or the equipment. They felt isolated in their shock, but on returning a few hours later were able to take more interest in the surroundings. Words most commonly used when referring to the NICU were 'shock,' 'surprise,' 'fright' and 'amazement' at the environment.

With reference to their own baby the most commonly used expressions indicated 'shock at his size,' 'difficulty in believing he was theirs,' 'pity,' 'love,' 'worry,' and 'relief' that the baby was actually alive.

This telling comment was made by the mother (a trained midwife) of the smallest baby in the survey (625 g):

I saw only her foot in the delivery room so it was hard to believe she was breathing. I was terrified they would dispose of her before I could get up to the nursery. It was hard to know what the paediatrician meant when he came back and said she was doing as well as could be expected. I waited until my husband came — I couldn't go alone. The head box was very frustrating. She almost fitted in it and it's very difficult to visualise a person when you can't see the head. Her eyes were closed, they did not open for two weeks. I said to them, 'Don't torture her to make her live — no heroics — it's not fair she has to suffer.'

Several mothers made similar comments: 'Poor little thing, I had never seen anything like her, she was beautiful. I had not imagined a fully formed human inside me.' or 'He was all respirator and tubes. There was not much baby. I felt so sorry for him. It was a very upsetting time.'

The mother's reaction to the baby. At the first interview the mothers were asked to describe their feelings toward the baby when they first saw him in NICU; their statements were later coded as positive, negative or mixed. They were also asked if those feelings had changed (see Fig. 7.1).

24 mothers had mixed feelings at first. In most of these cases the love these parents felt toward the baby was heavily over-shadowed by fear that a babe so small could not survive and that the treatment

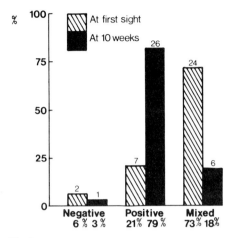

Fig. 7.1.

he was undergoing would prove too much for him. Three couples with previous neonatal losses feared not only for the baby but also for themselves, wondering how they would cope with another loss. They were somewhat reluctant, therefore, to allow themselves to love this child. Four mothers were given very pessimistic views by well-meaning relatives, friends and obstetricians. They felt themselves to be at a 'disadvantage' and had to 'overcome' this before being able to accept the optimism of the paediatricians. The majority managed to feel hopeful by the time the baby was doing well without life supports and 26 women felt positively about the baby by approximately 10 weeks. Two out of three who reported that the baby's eyes were not open when they first saw him/her were still in the 'mixed feelings' group at 10 weeks. Perhaps this delay of eye-contact had hampered the bonding process.

On the positive side, two mothers were almost unrealistic in their optimism. One stated she knew 'he would be okay because she loved him.' The other looked out of the window while the doctor talked about the problem: 'I don't need to know all that.'

Feedings. Feeding was discussed at length during both interviews as this, and weight gain, are of utmost importance to parents. It would seem that until they are convinced the baby can take milk they remain anxious about his survival. Feeding and love appear closely allied at the time of birth. As one mother commented, 'I did not express (my milk) although I had breast-fed five other children. It did not feel safe to love this baby, being so prem.' In normal full-term births, the infant licks and nuzzles the nipple and within an hour of birth he/she is commonly sucking vigorously. This is part of the reciprocal interaction that forms maternal attachment (Klaus & Kennell, 1982). The majority of the mothers were anxious to breast-feed. When asked at the first interview how they were intending to feed the baby, most started off by saying 'I was intending to breast-feed but ...' and then went on to relate the method currently being used.

Expressed breast milk (EBM). 26 mothers (79%) expressed their breast milk in the first weeks. By 10 weeks 13 of those (50%) were still expressing, one continuing for 27 weeks (see Fig. 7.2). Five felt persuaded to express the breast milk and one against doing so. The latter commented, 'I wanted to breast-feed but all the staff (at country hospital 200 miles from the city) and my doctor said the baby was too small and advised me not to express.' At 5–6 months of age when these babies weighed 3000–4500 g, seven (21%) were fully breast-fed and two half breast- and half bottle-fed.

15 mothers made comments relating to the specific procedures and feeding problems as they saw them. The majority of women felt very strongly about the value of expressing and about the breast milk itself. Some complained staff made unthinking remarks like, 'Is that all?' when a great deal of effort had gone into obtaining even small amounts. They felt such remarks and attitudes to be unhelpful. Others were upset on reading cot-side charts that their baby was receiving a formula when they had believed he was receiving the

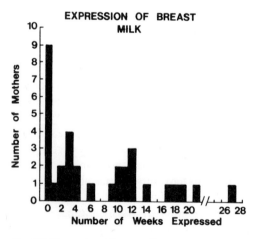

Fig. 7.2. Expression of breast milk

milk they had expressed. One woman stated, 'I was surprised when he was given formula. This was a worry because I knew the EBM (expressed breast milk) was nearly twice his daily needs.' One mother did not like her baby having EBM when it was not her own. She was not expressing, and perhaps this added to her current feeling of inadequacy and helplessness. Several women were happy to donate their excess EBM to other babies but all would have appreciated a little more personal discussion about this at the time.

Parents felt the ultimate method of feeding was their own decision and 81% were satisfied with their choices. Those who ultimately succeeded in fully breast feeding wished they had been given more information but were grateful, nevertheless, for the help they did receive. All of them took several weeks after baby's discharge from hospital to establish lactation fully. One comment from a mother whose baby was discharged at 19 weeks illustrates this:

> It took nearly 3 months to fully establish her on the breast. Some mothers would be horrified at how often I fed her. Sometimes it was every hour. Finally, she settled to 3 hourly feedings and is a happy contented baby now.

Parents felt additional information was needed about the establishment of breast feeding, increasing the supply, types of pumps and storing and freezing of milk.

The needs of mothers

Questions were aimed at discovering the parents' understanding of information and its usefulness to them regarding such issues as the baby's progress, hospital procedures and services arranged for their needs.

Information and explanation. Information was given to parents on their baby's progress by the paediatricians and nursing staff throughout the nursery stay. They were encouraged to ask questions and 75% did so; however, they frequently waited to ask a particular staff member with whom they felt more comfortable. The level of understanding varied with individuals, as did their need for knowledge. One mother commented, 'having some nursing experience was a mixed blessing. I almost understood, but I made my husband ask as I didn't want to look silly. It was all a bit high-powered for me.' Another mother said, 'I believed them. He would survive, but I can't see how he can be quite normal in his lungs' — and yet another avoided information altogether, 'they kept telling me things. I just knew he would be all right and I didn't want to know all those things.'

However, the majority wanted more information, especially about the effects of jaundice and anaemia. Four wanted to be informed about day to day events; for example, one parent wished she had been told about the precise starting time of her baby's exchange transfusion. She would have felt better if she had been praying for her baby at that time, rather than being comfortably in bed asleep.

Privacy in hospital. The mothers were asked how they felt about their hospital accommodation. The majority appeared satisfied with their environment. However, 16 of the 27 women in four bed bays with mothers of normal infants felt that all mothers with babies in NICU should be in the same ward. Four would have liked to have been offered a private room. Many said the ideal to them would have been a bed beside the baby.

Six mothers shared a room with another woman who had had a premature baby. They felt the support they were able to give one another to be mutually beneficial. Being with others in the same situation would obviate returning to the general postnatal ward area where women with full-term infants would perhaps find their sadness upsetting. Those who returned to the antenatal areas were concerned for the feelings of undelivered women, but felt it was good to be with old acquaintances.

Photographs. It is hospital practice to take colour photographs of each baby in NICU on the first day of life. Of the 28 mothers who received photographs, 12 felt it would have been better if they had received the photograph earlier, i.e. before arriving at NICU for the first time. Fathers who visited the baby before their wives often took the photo to her. The majority of parents felt it was important to receive the photograph as soon as possible after the infant left the delivery room. One mother said it was the only thing that saved her sanity. All parents were delighted with the pictures and many considered they formed a vital link, helping them accept the baby as a reality.

Visiting and telephone enquiries. Parents are encouraged to visit or telephone at any time. For obvious reasons parents from the country visited less often than those from the metropolitan area, although travelling from outer suburbs was often difficult, particularly for those without cars. 15 parents rang daily and four more frequently while babies were still in the NICU. The majority felt that phone enquiries were satisfactorily answered. However, parents whose private paediatricians telephoned to give routine reports were often alarmed by the call, especially when they had not been warned in advance that this was the doctor's normal routine. 'I heard, "It's Doctor X here" and I thought — she's dead — I had to call my husband; when he came off the phone it took a while for my husband to convince me she was okay. If the paediatrician had warned us that it was his habit to phone it would have been all right.'

Preparation for going home without the baby. The majority of mothers were very upset and felt enormous grief when leaving the baby in hospital. They felt the instructions they were given at the time of discharge regarding expression of breast milk, visiting and the like were inadequate. However, nearly half admitted they were so distressed they did not hear exactly what was said, 'I'm sure we were told things we forgot because once we were in the car I cried all the way; my poor husband, I don't know how he drove the 200 miles home.' Six months felt the staff could have repeated the instructions relating to EBM and given them a little more encouragement to increase the milk supply at the first few visits after going home. One mother described it thus: 'It is awful to go home without the baby. You need to keep busy. You mope about the house crying. You express, you bring the milk to the hospital and visit the baby. You need to be reminded of all the things you were going to do ... prepare the baby's room, etc.'

Those mothers referred from long distances for the delivery of premature infants felt particularly upset when they were fit to go home. The needs of other family members, who sometimes had already been left for weeks or months, also had to be considered. One mother mentioned feeling guilty about this, 'I felt guilty about being away from the other two children for so long (6 weeks). I felt guilty leaving him here. At home I felt guilty about the time spent expressing. When we don't visit I feel guilty and when we drag the others down here at weekends it's no fun for them. In fact, there's no end to my guilt.' However, in spite of feeling guilty at every turn, this particular mother coped with the situation extremely well. Guilt feelings among mothers who give birth prematurely are well documented (Klaus & Kennel, 1982).

Getting to know the baby. Many parents found it difficult to touch such small babies: 'I wanted to touch her, but I was too frightened. The sister helped me the next day and it was okay after that. I couldn't wait to hold her but when the time came, I was shaking.' and 'The first time we held her she was still attached to all those things. It was scary but wonderful — she looked right at me!'

Parents were asked if they felt their visits helped the baby. 18 saw their visits as beneficial to both themselves and the baby and felt the baby knew they were there even before he responded. 'Visiting is part of our treatment. We need to see her and she needs to see us. We are both sure she knows us. She has known our touch for weeks.'

Eight visited for their own sake and remarked that the baby did not worry who was there; 'We needed to *see* we had a son; I don't think he knows.' Five did not know if their visiting made any difference to the baby or not.

Parents were very pleased that they were encouraged to visit at all times and for as long as they wished. It also pleased them to be able to take grandparents and siblings into the nursery. They understood and approved that these visitors came one at a time and most felt these visits to be beneficial to the whole family. Only a few felt 'in the way' in NICU.

By approximately 10 weeks, most were able to hold him/her regularly. All but three stated their baby now knew them and they visited for longer periods as a consequence. Parents' visits ranged from twice a day to once a week and time spent varied from 1–8 hours.

Major anxieties

Baby's weight. 21 mothers were anxious about weight and used it as a major indicator of well being. Several kept a chart at home and celebrated every gain and were upset if a loss occurred.

Life supports. Ten mothers were worried by the removal of life supports and monitoring systems. Four remarked that staff gave as a reason for removing apnoea mattresses, for instance, that 'other babies needed them.' They would rather have heard that their particular infant was ready to do without.

Oxygen. The medical jargon used to describe oxygen usage confused many mothers. Three stated they just did not understand. A bewildered mother said, 'at one stage he was in a head box and they said it was good to be in 45% oxygen. I didn't know at the time oxygen was in the air we breathe, so it sounded a lot to me. It took weeks to get it sorted out so that I understood what was going on.'

Medical set-backs. 19 babies (57%) had 'set-backs'. They were transferred back to NICU or to another hospital for surgery, such as litigation of a patent ductus arteriosis or herniorrhaphy. Most of these babies returned a few days after surgery.

Nursery moves. In this institution it is practice 'to promote' babies from nursery to nursery as they improve and grow until they reach the last one, from which they will go home. The parents understood this system and were obviously upset when their baby was moved back to a previous area. There were a few occasions when parents felt that their baby was not ready for promotion and feared that by going to another nursery he would not come under sufficient observation.

Staff. Changing paediatricians upset parents more than rotation of nursing personnel. The chief comment was that doctors did not hand over properly and in some cases did not say they were moving on. Parents seen by the social worker felt they had been helped by this contact. None was critical of the staff's professional care, but several mentioned unthinking remarks, such as calling the baby 'it': 'I know it's hard to remember the baby's name when there are so many, but somehow a wrong sex is better than "it".' was how one mother expressed this complaint.

Preparation for taking baby home. The hospital attempts to teach care-giving skills at a level appropriate to each parent's needs.

Care-giving during visits. Nappy changes were frequently the first task at which parents became adept. Many were also pleased to assist with lavage feeding and by the time the baby was ready to go home the majority had fed him/her by breast or bottle during the preceding weeks.

Progress to total care-giving. In final preparation for baby's discharge four mothers were readmitted to a postnatal ward for rooming in and stayed for 48 hours. Five families stayed for 48 hours in a hospital flat from which it was easy for mother to attend the nursery every feed. Only one such flat is available and the demand is so great that only those families who live a considerable distance from the hospital are eligible to use it. Six mothers and babies were discharged to residential aftercare at one of the baby homes for 2–14 days. Four were transferred to country hospitals where mother could be accommodated or live close enough to spend all day caring for the baby. The remainder visited the nursery daily, staying 4–16 hours, giving total care in an area set aside for this purpose. All mothers were pleased that they had given baby's first bath in the hospital and for the time spent under supervision, although some felt they needed more time in these activities. In spite of preparation, for most parents, the actual day of homecoming was a shock. They thought that day would never come: 'I had so many things to do and I was so scared. I didn't know which way to turn. I felt like saying, "you'll have to keep her for another week until I get organised".' One woman felt staff should take more responsibility here: 'Mothers need reminding actively to prepare for the occasion; for example, have all the nappies and clothes ready, read up on increasing the milk supply, prepare some casseroles and meals which can be deep-frozen, make contact with the local clinic or nursing mothers group; then when the day is "on" you know which people to contact for help.'

Several mothers were told not to forget he or she 'needs stimulation' without any explanation of what was meant by this: 'I was told he needed stimulation. I don't know if he should have exercises or massage or what? I've got a university degree and I feel I should understand, but they don't say what they mean. I'm very worried because I've done nothing about it. Some of the other mothers would not understand either.'

Corrected age. It was important that parents had a good understanding of the implications of the term 'corrected age' so that they were not unrealistic in their expectations of their child's developmental skills.

Age is generally measured from conception, so that if a baby is born 12 weeks before his expected date of delivery he is presumed to be about 12 weeks behind his full-term peers in reaching certain developmental milestones. Put more simply, a 6-month-old premature baby who was 12 weeks early would be expected to be at approximately the same developmental level as a full-term 3-month child — therefore, 3 months is his 'corrected age'.

Parents needed to appreciate that the premature infant has to make up the development he missed in the uterus and for this reason such babies usually lag behind in growth and development, compared with the term infant, for the first 2 years of life.

At home

20 mothers felt the need to seek advice during the first week at home. The majority found their baby hard to settle after feeds. It appeared they cried more at night and suffered more 'colic' than other babies. Several wished they had been warned of this. The babies were between 12 and 20 weeks old when they did go home and weighed between 3000 and 5000 g.

Ten parents said they had experienced difficulties with relatives and acquaintances and casual 'pram peepers': 'I was in the supermarket and a woman said "what a little dear, how old is he?" I said, "7 months." She looked at me oddly and said, "Can't be yours, looks more like 7 weeks." That really upset me. People don't understand. After that I lied about his age.'

Several felt 'corrected age' and public disbelief about size and age needed more careful explanation.

Follow-up

17 mothers kept appointments at hospital paediatric clinics within 4 weeks of the babe's discharge.

12 mothers with private consultant paediatricians were seen between 4 and 16 weeks after leaving the hospital. Nine of these mothers would have liked an earlier appointment. The general feeling was that the consultant paediatrician should be interested in normal progress and advise on aspects of concern to the mother even though he may consider such worries to be trivial. If consultant paediatricians are unable to see mothers at short notice, it would help parents to have more explanation and referrals to general practitioners and hospital-outpatient clinics for minor emergencies, out of hours advice and routine management.

Mothers who lived at a distance and who did not return to paediatric clinics all stated they had ready access to general practitioners or their family doctors. 17 mothers were visited by domiciliary midwifery sisters attached to the hospital and one was visited by the district nurse after discharge from a country hospital. Everyone found these visits helpful. Those who rang the hospital nursery appreciated the help and reassurance received.

At the time of the second interview, 25 (75%) mothers were attending Infant Welfare Centres and only two felt the Infant Welfare Sister had not had enough experience with premature babies to be helpful to them.

Parents support group

The group meets every 2 weeks, alternating between day and evening sessions, on a fortnightly basis. Most parents approved of the usefulness of such a group; of those surveyed only five couples had attended before 10 weeks and only two came back after going home.

Fathers

It is in comparatively recent times that fathers have become closely involved with antenatal preparation, birth and caring for infants. The birth of a premature baby also comes as a shock to the father, who is equally unprepared for the event. Even when the NICU is in the same building as the delivery room he may still be suffering from the effects of a dash through traffic along an unfamiliar route. Fathers' reactions to NICU were similar to those of the mother: 'I was shocked when I first went to NICU and things left me numb. I just couldn't talk about it.'

Although more fathers noticed other babies and took more interest in the machines on their first visit, only four of 14 who visited the NICU before their wives were able to give their wives any useful information. Several made statements to the effect, 'I didn't want to frighten my wife. I was so shocked; she was so small' or 'the paediatrician explained everything, but I was in a state of shock looking at the baby and I didn't hear what he said.'

In many cases the father's comments agreed with those made by their wives.

One father of a previous premature baby said, 'It is our second time here. William was 31 weeks, so I did find Mark (27 weeks) easier to accept. The worst was when he needed the respirator after 4 days. Men need to cry too. One of the sisters was great, but the doctor couldn't take it,' and another who was a first-time father: 'I thought she would be the only one. What a surprise to see all those other babies, so small and perfect. I used to check on some of the smaller ones each day and always looked at the before and after photos.'

The nursery had several large notice boards covered with photos of babies at all stages from one with father's wedding ring on his wrist to teenagers. More fathers than mothers mentioned this gallery of photographs and were particularly helped by the second, third and subsequent photos added over the years.

14 fathers were present at the birth. Nine waited outside the delivery room, including five Caesarean births. Although most parents had briefly seen the baby in the delivery room, it was more likely to be the father who first saw the baby in NICU.

Nine of 14 fathers who visited before their wives remained closely involved with the baby, taking an active part in care-giving and continued to do so at home.

Two fathers were more confident than their wives that their babies recognised them from a very early age: 'She knew me that first night and she always knows me when I come.'

Several fathers noticed staff attitudes and marvelled at them: 'I was looking through the glass to the next room and the nurse was talking to the babies and really loving the one she was feeding. There were no parents in the room — they sure don't do it for the money.'

There were several very angry remarks made by fathers in regard to obstetricians and paediatricians. Perhaps they were better able to express this than their wives, for example: 'He (the obstetrician) had no business to book my wife into a hospital with no NICU facility. When he put in the cervical stitch he must have known it could be a premature birth.'

DISCUSSION

Crisis of premature birth

Prematurity poses special problems for newborn infants and parents alike. These problems need the expertise of many disciplines. In the NICU parents should be involved, informed, able to question and have access to knowledge appropriate to their personal needs in order for them to feel part of the infant's care from birth. All childbirth produces anxiety; the premature birth much more than average as parents are unable to cope alone and unresolved anxiety may lead to a poor mother-child relationship (Kaplan, 1960).

Family's emotional experience of premature birth

Premature birth is a crisis for most parents which they will approach individually in ways that reflect their personality and past and present experiences. Regardless of the form this takes, there appears to be no movement towards resolution until the infant is at 40 weeks of gestational age, about which time he is able to interact with his parents (Klaus & Kennell, 1976). Many of our mothers were still feeling anxious and stressed at the second interview, so obviously for them the crisis had not resolved. For some, their crisis of prematurity started before the birth when premature labour threatened and they were admitted to hospital, several up to 3 months prior to the birth; during this time the family was disrupted by the separation, and yet appeared to be managing very well without the mother. This did not help her confidence; she missed them and they did not appear to need her. The mother forced to spend time in hospital is in need of a morale-booster and instead she comes to deliver a small, unattractive baby which is 'like an emotional slap in the face,' as one mother put it.

There was a remarkable consistency about the feeling of shock that this scrap of humanity, with all his tubes and wires, is in fact their child. Many of the babies in the survey were at or under 28 weeks, before which time they were unable to give signals to which parents can respond (Minde et al, 1978). There were several infants under 27 weeks gestation. Most of these had their eyes closed for the first week or so of life, and in consequence parent-infant interaction was delayed (Klaus & Kennell, 1982) from lack of eye-to-eye contact. It is understandable that these parents felt a sense of loss and grief as they had not reached the stage in pregnancy when self-interest changes to a primary concern for the unborn baby (Taylor & Hall, 1979).

Fathers also suffered emotionally during the time of crisis but it would appear that because of the early contact with the infant they often became attached to their premature child (Minde, 1980) and continued to be involved in care-giving at home. There was a long period of adjustment to be made; for these parents the length of time and the type of help needed was individual.

Information and education

Throughout both interviews the needs of parents for information was apparent. The majority had their questions answered but it appeared that most felt the language used was too complex or that they needed to be told several times. Individuals have widely varying needs and levels of understanding. Professionals should recognise this and in talking with the parents, and not at them, should assess their needs and communicate accordingly. One might ask why we continue to use medical jargon when it is unintelligible to most parents and even to many professionals from other specialities. Most parents have a need to be informed but there are the minority who do not wish for too many details and accept meagre information without question, possibly as a means of coping with an otherwise overwhelming situation. It is equally important that people in this category are not worried with facts they do not seek. On the other hand, there is a real need to spend time with parents in order to reach reliable conclusions about their needs in this area.

Misunderstandings

When people are ill, anxious and confused, it is not surprising that sometimes there are misunderstandings of medical advice; however, the extent of misunderstanding in this group was surprisingly high. For example, some mothers had regarded the insertion of a cervical suture as being a guarantee that the pregnancy would be full term. Another mother felt her doctor did not regard her seriously when she reported the draining of liquor amni; she felt she was treated as though she were unable to recognise and describe her own symptoms and feelings. Misunderstandings occurred because of lack of knowledge of the gestational age at which a baby can survive; some mothers misunderstood statements about 'termination' of their pregnancy and did not expect a live birth. This type of misunderstanding was probably also a factor in their understanding of 'in labour' transfer; these transfers were upsetting to parents who believed they were having an abortion or miscarriage. Such confusions add to the anxiety and can cause resentment and mistrust of the professional care, and in no way prepared the parents for the reality of a very small premature baby.

A labour described by the mother as painful and distressing did not appear to have any effect on the relationship with the babies in the long-term. The fact that they were given 'false or misleading' (their words) information about prematurity, their labour, or survival prospects for the baby, did not appear to make the labour more of a problem to several and this in turn made them more fearful of their first visit to NICU.

Mothers of term babies have problems with 'false, misleading' or lack of information and conflicting advice (Cartwright, 1979), and the mother of the premature infant is even less able to cope with the situation.

Development

The course of development of premature babies was a source of puzzlement to the majority of these parents and the term 'corrected age' or 40 weeks of gestational age needed careful explanation. When provided with this information they were more able to view their child's progress realistically and resist making comparisons with full-term infants.

Stimulation

Several parents stated that they had been told their baby needed 'stimulation' when they went home. This was poorly understood and needed to be illustrated with examples of the type of activities envisaged.

More written information

Several requests were made for books about prematurity and with particular attention to feeding the premature baby including the storage, freezing and expressing of breast milk; skin contact and/or massage for premature babies; stimulation; jaundice and anaemia. It is interesting that the two medical conditions causing the most concern, and about which the parents needed more information regarding the future are both, medically, minor complications, easily treated. Perhaps it is significant; both jaundice and anaemia can be seen by looking at the baby. As parents are reassured as the baby gains weight — so they are upset if the colour is not 'right'.

Difficult behaviour at home

To professionals, the problem very low birthweight infants have with 'colic,' night wakefulness, periodic crying, feeding problems and generally unsettled behaviour are not surprising. The NICU and the subsequent nurseries are full of light and noise day and night, totally ignoring human sleeping rhythms. Incubator noise alone is considerable and some nurseries play taped background music. It is not surprising these babies find the dark quiet nights at home somewhat alarming. Parents need a lot of patience in understanding that they may suffer many sleepless nights in order to train these babies to sleep at night and join the mainstream of the human race. Easy access to advice and counselling services are important to parents. Parent support groups as reported by Shosenberg (1980) are helpful to some during the baby's hospitalization, but many seem unable to partake in group activities until much later. For some the 'one to one' counselling situation is more appropriate.

IMPLICATIONS FOR NURSING PRACTICE

Facilities

The recent improvements and innovations in the care of parents associated with NICU have been appreciated, but further thought for their feelings is indicated and further facilities are needed, even in units considered by professionals to be centres of excellence. Among these facilities either appreciated or requested are the following:

Access to baby at all times
Beds for parents either in unit or as near as possible
Photographs of babies as soon as possible
Mothers' room in the unit with day beds, comfortable chairs with

tea and coffee-making facilities

Pre-school day care centre for siblings

Parking for motor cars, either free or subsidized. (You can't feed a meter if you're feeding a baby!)

Pay telephone for parent use in or near the nurseries

Social worker, available also at weekends and evenings

Education for parents in care-giving, with attention to: instruction, both written and practical, in expressed breast milk and breast feeding a premature baby; practical demonstrations of milk formulae and bathing the baby; family planning advice; and encouragement to parents to form support groups.

Action

The aim of improving all the services to parents may be helped by attention to the following:

Escort available to parents as soon as practical after the birth, even from the delivery room if this is possible, as well as during the next few days until mother is well, and feels sufficiently confident to find her own way to the nursery.

A photograph of every baby on admission to NICU to be given to the mother as soon as possible, with the invitation to come herself to visit.

Encourage parents to name their baby, and display the given name on the cot for use at all times.

Encourage parents to touch and talk to their baby as soon as they are ready. Staff should be sensitive to the parents' wishes in this matter.

Staff who do not work in NICU but who care for mothers should be informed of the baby's condition so they can have meaningful discussions with the mother.

If mothers wish to express breast milk, they need help and encouragement from both ward and nursery staff, with information about the system used for collection, storage and delivery to the baby. Constant encouragement is needed to keep the supply when she leaves the hospital and the instructions need to be explained several times. The occasional misunderstanding or mishap with EBM should be mentioned. Alternative formulae to be used in the absence of EBM should also be provided. Information on increasing the supply and re-lactation before mothers' discharge from hospital would be helpful for many.

Encourage mothers to actively prepare for the baby's homecoming; assist by building the mother's confidence to cope with the baby at home. Ensure she is adept at care-giving skills and praise her performance of these tasks.

Advise on whom to call and where to go for counselling and follow-up services in the community and the hospital.

Solicit help from parents to keep a 'gallery' or notice board of 'before and after' pictures.

If the mother is in another hospital or unable to visit, contact should be maintained by photographs, letters from the baby (Eager, 1977), and phone calls. If the parents are to be telephoned by nurse or doctor with routine progress reports, they should be informed this is to happen to save them from 'fearing the worst' every time the phone rings!

Acknowledgements

The survey described here was supported by the Department of Obstetrics and Gynaecology of the University of Melbourne and the Royal Women's Hospital.

Grateful acknowledgement is made to Dr W.H. Kitchen, Director of Paediatrics, and to Mrs M.N. Ryan; Research Fellow to this department. For the help of nursery staff and colleagues, many thanks and we are indebted to the parents who took part.

An article based on this survey was published in Australian Nurses Journal, December/January, 1981.

REFERENCES

Budin P 1907 The Nursling. Caxton, London
Cartwright A 1979 The dignity of labour — A study of childbearing and induction. Tavistock, London
Congalton A A 1969 Status and prestige in Australia. Cheshire, Melbourne
Eager M 1977 Long distance nurturing of the family bond. American Journal of Maternal Child Nursing 2: 293–294
Kaplan D M, Mason E A 1960 Maternal reactions to premature birth viewed as an acute emotional disorder. American Journal Orthopsychiatry 30: 539–552
Kitchen W H, Ryan M M, Rickards A, McDougall A B, Billson F A, Keir E H, Naylor F D 1980 A longitudinal study of very low birthweight infants. IV. An overview of performance at 8 years of age. Developmental Medicine and Child Neurology 22: 172–188
Klaus M H, Fanaroff A A 1979 Care of the high risk neonate, 2nd edn. Saunders, Philadelphia
Klaus M H, Kennell J H 1976 Maternal-infant bonding, Mosby, St Louis
Klaus M H, Kennell J H 1982 Parent-infant bonding, Mosby, St Louis
Mangurten H H, Slade C, Fitzsimonds D 1979 Parent support in the care of high risk newborns. Journal of Obstetric Gynecologic and Neonatal Nursing 8: 275–277

Minde K K 1980 Bonding of parents to premature infants — Theory and practice. In: Taylor P M (ed) Parent-infant relationships. Monographs in Neonatology. Grune and Stratton, New York, ch 14, p 291–309

Minde K K, Trehub S, Corter C, Boukydis Celhoffer L, Marton P 1978 Mother-child relationships in the premature nursery. An observational study. Pediatrics 61: 373–379

Taylor P M, Hall B L 1979 Parent-infant bonding: Problems and opportunities in a perinatal centre. Seminars in Perinatology 3:1, 73–75

Yu V Y H, Jamison J, Astbury J 1981 Parents reactions to unrestricted parental contact with infants in the intensive care nursery. The Medical Journal of Australia 1:294–296

Postpartum depression

The postpartum experience, occurring in the period following child-birth, is characterized by numerous adaptations necessary for the woman to restore her physical, emotional, and social health. The postpartum woman is involved in an adaptation cycle working towards a healing and restorative process. This adaptation cycle demands an interplay between the woman's metabolic and psychic energies. The physiological adaptations required after childbirth are widely recognized. However, healthy adaptations in the postpartum period demand an interface between a women's physical and her psychosocial well-being. Thus, the cognitive, affective, and social transitions are also considered to be of equal importance as the physiological changes occurring in the postpartum period.

This chapter to address the phenomenon of postpartum depression will be organized as follows:

1. The process by which a woman adapts her life in the period following childbirth (known as postpartum adaptation) will be conceptually described.

2. The scope of the problem relative to postpartum depression will be identified.

3. A theoretical perspective will be presented for two areas: (a) depression theories in general and (b) theories specifically related to postpartum depression.

4. Clinical mainfestations will be identified and explained in terms of their functional significance.

5. Onset and duration of depressive symptomatology in postpartum women will be discussed.

6. The influencing variables will be listed as identified in the current literature.

7. Women's vulnerability to postpartum depression will be discussed in terms of findings from a research project.

8. Nursing assessment will be discussed relative to two processes:

(a) differentiation between postpartum blues versus postpartum depression, and (b) early case finding for symptomatology suggestive of postpartum depression.
  9. Nursing therapeutic strategies will be identified and discussed.

POSTPARTUM ADAPTATION

The postpartum period was once viewed as a time of tranquil recuperation, anticlimactic to the excitement and suspense surrounding labour and birth. However, many authors eventually began to describe the postpartum period as a time when the real drama associated with childbirth was just beginning. Caplan (1959) articulated a psychodynamic perspective on postpartum adaptation, and emphasized a disequilibrium that occurs in the woman's ego boundaries making the woman vulnerable to psychological stress. Caplan viewed the postpartum period as a time when a woman was particularly vulnerable to emotional crises because her energy reserves could be rapidly depleted by such factors as fatigue, effects from medications, length of labour, difficulties in the delivery process, and fears or concerns associated with the events in pregnancy and childbirth. Rubin (1961) conceptualized the postpartum woman as in transition between a state of dependency and independency. Rubin described two phases, labeled as 'taking-in' and 'taking-hold,' which provide behavioral cues of the woman's progression from dependency states toward independency. LeMasters (1965) described the postpartum period as a crisis-provoking time because the addition of a new child forced the couple and their family to realign their interpersonal relationships from a dual, pair-type organizational structure to a triadic-plus communication system. Thus, LeMasters conceptualized parenthood as a maturational crisis that peaked during the postpartum period. Affonso (1977) introduced the concept of 'missing pieces' as part of a cognitive task for the integration of the entire childbirth experience as a meaningful, whole, life event. A woman's construal that selected 'pieces' of her childbirth experience were missing served the functional purpose of facilitating data collection from the environment such that the woman could then piece the many events into a meaningful cognitive and affective sequence, similar to the completion of a puzzle. Affonso stressed that the process of cognitive mapping out of the childbirth experience should occur during the first 6 weeks of the postpartum period and is a significant psychological task for the woman in terms of maintaining future mental and emotional health. Women who did not engage in cognitive mapping of their childbirth experience due to 'missing pieces' reported emotional and mental distress, some for many years duration (Affonso, 1977). Clark (1979) highlighted the postpartum woman as being in a 'woman to motherhood' transitional phase. Clark described the postpartum woman as having to deal with many critical issues, such as resolving unmet expectations versus reality, letting go of perceived losses, and reorganization of multiple roles involving career versus parenting goals. Thus, the postpartum woman is forced to find a balance between events occurring in her life that have the potential for ambivalence and conflicts (such as experiencing both the joys and frustrations of parenting). Another author (Mercer, 1981) expanded the concept of postpartum adaptation by emphasizing the importance of the many social transitions that are involved in childbearing. A woman's social sphere may become constricted during pregnancy and make her vulnerable to feelings of alienation and isolation. Mercer brought new meaning to commonly seen behaviors in postpartum women such as frequent story-telling, telephone contacts, desires to share pictures and tape recordings of the birth experience. Such behaviors are functional as they provide an acceptable modality by which the woman can re-establish and expand her social contacts in the adult world after childbirth. Decreased social contacts have been found to correlate with depressive symptomatology in postpartum women (Oakley, 1980; Affonso, 1982). The cognitive and affective changes that can accompany the physiologic transitions inherent in the postpartum period have also been described (Kane, 1968). Examples of such changes include increased tension; irritability; somatic disturbances such as palpitations, tremulousness, and shortness of breath; labile mood; increased sleepiness; fatigue, self-depressive thinking; diminished mental alertness manifested through inability to maintain attention, difficulty in recall of events, and frustrations in performing simple manual tasks. Such broad and non-specific changes closely resemble the disruptions observed in mood and thought processes which accompany various forms of psychopathology (Cameron, 1963). The imposition of these cognitive-affective disturbances may disrupt the woman's healthy functioning and precipitate defensive, neurotic behavioral styles. The neurotic behavioral symptoms which are likely to manifest after childbirth have been described as increased anxiety rapidly escalating to panic proportions, obsession with fear of abandonment, phobias, and depressive symptomatology (Kaij & Nilsson, 1972).

A common theme of most authors who have developed a conceptual perspective on the postpartum period is that this period is a time of tremendous transitions and adaptations. The upheaval of psychosocial adaptations amid the unavoidable physiological transitions in the maternal reproductive-hormonal systems, makes the postpartum woman especially vulnerable to disruptions in daily activities leading to emotional instability and decreased socializations. Thus, the postpartum period is presently accepted as a time of vulnerability to psychological stress and emotional crises for many childbearing women (Caplan, 1959).

POSTPARTUM DEPRESSION: SCOPE OF THE PROBLEM

The most common psychopathological process to occur in the postpartum period is depression (Hamilton, 1962; Pitt, 1968). Depressive conditions are reported to account for approximately 50–60% of the disturbances manifested in the postpartum period (Bardon, 1972). The reported incidence rates of postpartum depression vary widely, between 3% and 27% in selected samples of childbearing women (Pitt, 1968; Clarke & Williams, 1979; Manly et al, 1982). For many years postpartum depression was not considered to be a major obstetrical or mental health problem, possibly because the emphasis after childbirth was primarily on the restoration of the maternal reproductive-hormonal systems. However, since the last decade, many studies have reported the increased occurrence of depressive symptomatology in women after childbirth (Bardon, 1972; Cone, 1972; Liakos et al, 1972; Tod, 1972; Manly et al, 1982). Thus, modern obstetrical books now state that depressive symptoms which complicate postpartum adaptation do constitute an obstetric morbidity problem (Pritchard & MacDonald, 1980; Danforth, 1982). The scope of the problem has been articulated: '... it would appear that a sizeable minority of women is vulnerable to depression following childbirth.' (Manly et al, 1982).

THEORETICAL PERSPECTIVE

Depression in general

To gain a better understanding of postpartum depression, it is imperative to have an overview of the theoretical perspectives on depression in general. The following is a brief summation of the various theories in the literature.

Clinical depression is distinguished from normal reactions of grief and sadness in terms of its severity, duration or persistence, and effects on the individual's day to day functioning. Clinically significant depression is generally categorized by disturbances in five dimensions: (1) moods initially become labile and move toward an apathetic, despondent nature; (2) thought processes change toward a negative construal of the world, self, and future; (3) interpersonal relationships deteriorate as a result of social and emotional withdrawal; (4) biological patterns are altered with increased somatic discomforts; (5) activity level is disturbed in terms of frequent lethargy and/or increased agitation and irritability (Arkowitz, 1980; Teuting et al, 1981).

There are several theoretical speculations regarding the phenomenon of depression. Psychoanalytic theory postulates that an individual has a predisposition to depression because of dependence upon external sources for ego support; upon actual or perceived loss of such sources, introjection of the loss object occurs and is accompanied by any unresolved guilt, hate, and negative affect associated with the loss experience (Freud, 1917). The behavioral perspective views depression as resulting from a low schedule of response-contingent positive reinforcement due to decreased reinforcers in the environment or that the person possesses inadequate social skills to emit behaviors that could be positively reinforced (Lewinsohn, 1975). The cognitive theory proposes that depressed individuals feel and behave as they do because of errors in their logical thinking that create a critical, negative cognitive set regarding how they view themselves, the world, and the future (Beck, 1967). The physiological perspective highlights biochemical alterations as generating depressive mood changes; specifically lower levels of the catecholamines, norepinephrine and serotonin, contribute to depressive symptomatology (Gallant & Simpson, 1976). A social perspective links the origin of depression to multiple factors intertwined with societal conditions such as environmental, political, economic, cultural influences (Brown & Harris, 1978). The day to day experiences of the depressed individual are disrupted because of social contingencies operating and thus, depression is not a problems only for the individual but a problem for society as well. An interactional/ interpersonal theoretical approach has also been developed. Coyne (1976) postulated that depression is a manifestation of disruption in the person's interaction patterns resulting from discrepancies between the behaviors emitted and the social responses elicited from others. The larger the discrepancies and the longer they persist, the more likely an individual will experience disruptions in cognitive, affective, and behavioral functioning which lead to depression.

Theories on postpartum depression

For many years a prominent theoretical perspective on the depression in women after childbirth was psychodynamic in nature. Explanations for depressive symptomatology in the postpartum period were related to such psychoanalytic concepts as perceived losses that create separation anxiety and panic, unresolved developmental conflicts that create ambivalence in present interpersonal relationships, and narcissistic identification with introjected hostility. The following are examples of explanations for the causes of postpartum depression, based on the works of Benedek (1970), Caplan (1959), and Deutsch (1944).

Dependent oral needs are revived during pregnancy and frustration of such needs, either self-imposed or by others, activates psychopathologic reactions of which anxiety and depression are prominent in childbearing women.

The psychologic state of pregnancy involves an inner-directed regressive tendency which causes mood disturbances; a calm elation of the narcissistic state can be replaced rapidly by an anxious depressive mood reflecting deep-seated insecurities.

The physiology of pregnancy brings about regression of ego allowing activation of impulses and the ego state of imbalance remains especially vulnerable in the postpartum period (Caplan, 1959).

Perceived losses of the symbiotic relationship with the fetus and the loss of the narcissistic state provided by pregnancy generates separation anxiety which lead to ambivalence in present relationships.

Pregnancy and the fetus serve as a natural source for the woman's fantasies which consist mainly of narcissistic libido charged with ambivalence. Depending upon what the fantasies represent, hope for fulfillment can occur after childbirth or there can be revival of hostility creating panic or depression.

Unresolved oedipal conflicts can create tensions in the woman's adjustment to the mothering role such that narcissistic identification with one's mother occurs with introjected hostility. Such identification is the primary, complicated interpersonal process Freud labeled as creating the symptoms seen in depressed persons.

The developmental events by which a woman's personality is organized, serves as important cues to her emotional adaptation after childbirth. A woman charged with frustrated dependency needs, separation anxiety, and ambivalence, is likely to experience postpartum depression.

The psychodynamic perspective has the strength of offering the most comprehensive, interesting, and elaborate explanations regarding the cause and development of postpartum depression. However, it also has the limitations of not providing a modality by which the theoretical constructs can be tested, and its psychotherapeutic strategies are expensive, demand a long-term course, and measurable outcomes are difficult to attain.

Another popular perspective is biological in nature, attributing depression in postpartum women to hormonal imbalances. Depressive symptomatology tends to peak early in the puerperium (third postpartum day) which is the same point in time when there is a precipitous drop in estrogen and progesterone levels due to the termination of placental functioning. (Dalton, 1971; Paykel et al, 1980) The hormones estrogen and progesterone are believed to influence moods, whereby estrogen levels activate extroverted behaviors and progesterone stimulate introversion. Thus, any imbalance between these two hormones can contribute to the mood swings typically seen in depressed postpartum women. The strength of the hormonal theory is that it allows depression to be attributed to biological factors which can easily be separated from a woman's psychological disposition. This permits a causal explanation that is more neutral and based on physical factors that are not so intimately interwined with the more personal aspects of a woman's personality and developmental history. The disadvantage of the biological theory is that in spite of its popularity with obstetrical health professionals, the hormonal hypothesis is insufficient, does not offer insights as to why depression does not necessarily subside when hormonal levels return to normal, nor does it explain why only selected women become clinically depressed after childbirth when all women undergo hormonal imbalances as a result of pregnancy (Manly et al, 1982). Also, the theory only offers an explanation for depressive symptomatology manifested during the first postpartum week. Thus, the current literature advocates expansion of other hypothesis to explain postpartum depression until more elaborate biochemical technologies can substantiate evidence for a definite relationship between hormonal levels and depressive symptomatology (Gelder, 1978; Steiner, 1979; Manly et al, 1982).

Currently, two other theoretical perspectives are emerging in the literature as attempts to explain the phenomena of postpartum depression. A social perspective proposes that women become depressed after childbirth due to social-environmental factors and thus, the problem is not an individual one but a societal concern. Examples of the undesirable social-environmental influences are: (1) lack of sufficient economic and political supports to maintain adequate housing, provide parenting, and meet health care needs (Brown & Harris, 1978); (2) inability to get relief from parenting activities, difficulties in resumption into the social adult world, and unrealistic myths about motherhood as reinforced by society through the mass media (Oakley, 1980); (3) a tendency for women to develop emotional dependency and attachment to others in meeting one's emotional needs, and frequent frustrations in attempts to meet such needs due to rapid changes in the social structure regarding women's roles (Scarf, 1980).

Another perspective is cognitive in nature and focuses on how a woman's thought processes influence her moods and behaviours. One study (Manly et al, 1982) proved negligible support for its original purpose of testing whether there was a relationship between depression and the attributional style of learned helplessness (as developed by Seligman, 1975), but advocated that cognitive factors played a prominent role in the development of depression in women after childbirth. This speculation was supported in another study that measured postpartum via a cognitive based assessment method and found significant correlations between selected cognitive factors and depression in women during the third and eighth postpartum weeks (Affonso, 1982).

For the present, the literature is inadequate in providing a satisfactory theoretical perspective on postpartum depression. Selected pieces from the differing theories are articulated well, but close examination of each perspective reveals that the state of the art regarding theory development is far from adequate. The emergence of new data from studies utilizing a cognitive-social conceptual model holds promise for progress in theory development for the phenomenon of postpartum depression.

CLINICAL MANIFESTATIONS

Postpartum depression is considered to be a multi-faceted, heterogeneous phenomenon, characterized by a behavioral repertoire which affects all levels of the woman's physical, psychological and social functioning. Postpartum depression is characterized by the presence of the following behaviors, not necessarily in the order presented or with every behavior manifested (see Table 8.1 for list of clinical manifestations).

Table 8.1 Clinical manifestations suggestive of postpartum depression

1. Mood disturbances escalate
2. Crying/tearfulness may or may not be present
3. Low frustration tolerance
4. Increased irritability and/or aggressiveness
5. Anger and/or hostility
6. Social and emotional withdrawal
7. Normal parenting tasks rapidly become a burden
8. Preoccupation or disinterest in the newborn
9. Cognitive changes/disturbances
10. Generalized fatigue and feeling 'all is not well'
11. Somatic disturbances interrupt daily functioning
12. Apathy and despondency

Mood disturbances escalate

Moods can easily become disturbed without a precipitating event. The lability in moods can span a wide range of affect (such as irritability, apathy, anger, despondency) lasts beyond a few days, and takes some time and effort for the woman to return to a state of emotional stability. Most women will express some awareness and concern that their 'moods and feelings are not the same as prior to pregnancy,' or that one's moods are 'not back to normal'. The mood swings may initially be reactive but over time cannot convert back to baseline such that the woman is viewed as always 'moody'.

Crying and tearfulness

There is the myth that the depressed postpartum woman is likely to manifest frequent crying or hystrionic-type behaviors. However, crying and tearfulness may or may not be present. Frequent crying suggest a state of hyper-emotional sensitivity (Derbolowsky et al, 1979). This 'hypersensitive emotional state' is initially communicated by crying and/or tearfulness and can be a precursor phase to postpartum depression if the hypersensitivity is not reduced to permit some degree of emotional stability. Thus, frequent crying or tearfulness is an early indicator of postpartum emotional distress. For women who do not exhibit crying or tearfulness, the early signs of distress may manifest in more vague behaviors such as low frustration, irritability or aggressiveness.

Low frustration tolerance

Simple responsibilities and tasks may easily trigger frustrated behavioral reactions especially in relation to parenting encounters. Frustrations begin to manifest in responses to events that were once sources of satisfaction and pleasure. Frequently the degree of frustrated reactions seem out of proportion to the precipitating event. Escalation of frustrations also signify some awareness that the woman is unable to resolve her emotional distress through her own resources and becomes increasingly frustrated every time she fails in her attempts to do so.

Increased irritability and/or aggressiveness

Irritation and unprovoked aggression ar early warning signs that a woman is vulnerable to postpartum depression. The reactive behaviors of being irritable and/or aggressive, with or without a precipitating event, communicates a level of awareness that the woman's life is not settling down into the expected, usual patterns after childbirth. The aggression is an attempt to mobilize energies to provoke an environmental response for help as the woman comes to grip with the realization that the discomforts of her present situation will not go away by themselves. Aggressive behaviors can be predicted to elicit a response from others, but typically they evoke negative reactions. Unfortunately, aggressive behaviors are not yet viewed as a plea for help due to the individual's inability to resolve the emotional distress on one's own. Aggressive behaviors also serve the function of allowing the woman to feel she can exert some control on external events as she struggles with the agony of losing control internally with her affect, thoughts, and behavioral reactions.

Anger and/or hostility

Anger has been described as one of the stages in the grief and grieving process (Kubler-Ross, 1969). The manifestation of angry behaviors is a healthy sign reflecting the woman's capability to respond with 'fighting spirit' in an attempt to improve her present situation. Unfortunately, the anger is frequently misconstrued as a negative, unfavourable response because of the stereotype that 'women should be happy and joyous after childbirth,' especially if the outcome is a physically healthy mother and baby. However, there are many legitimate aspects of the childbearing experience that a woman may be angry about if she is a mentally healthy adult. Examples are unmet expectations, role conflicts, increased responsibilities, altered social environments, and escalation of financial commitments (Clark & Affonso, 1979). Thus, angry behaviors can be a sign of an attempt to rectify an undesirable situation. However, if the angry energies are not worked through, defused, or channeled into constructive activities, then hostility sets in. Hostility is unresolved anger that has been internalized and may be discharged through projection upon the environment or turned upon the self. Hostility is more likely to be exhibited in interpersonal relationships. In essence, hostility rapidly evokes guilt and internalized excessive hostility remains a dangerous threat to the individual (Cameron, 1963). Thus, if anger is unresolved and the woman develops a new behavioral coping style of being hostile to self or others, the long-term consequences on her mental health can be grave. Hostility will be more difficult to resolve and frequently dictates assistance from structured therapeutic interventions.

Social and emotional withdrawal

One of the early signs suggestive that the postpartum woman is experiencing some depression is her gradual retreat from usual, expected interactive activities with family, relatives and friends. The birth of a baby activates numerous social and emotional encounters by which the childbirth event is shared, compared, and integrated. When a woman is unable to engage in normal patterns of interactions with others, the withdrawal behaviors acquire great significance during the postpartum period. Withdrawal behaviors can manifest very subtly and may go unnoticed because of the protective nature afforded by society to many women after childbirth, such as attributing lack of socializations to fatigue and the need for rest and recuperation. However, the manifestation and progression of the following behavioral reactions should be appreciated as warning signs that a withdrawal repertoire is operating and nurturing postpartum depression: frequent cancelled appointments, refusals to accept telephone contacts, disinterest in others and events in the environment, escalation of excuses for unkept social engagements, retreat into selected rooms or areas in the home and inability to attend to details occurring in daily routines.

Normal parenting tasks rapidly become a burden

Women who are experiencing healthy postpartal adaptation are able to respond to the normal trials and challenges of early parenting with some degree of successful outcomes. Healthy women may have an occasional depressive reaction to a parenting encounter that is posing some difficulties. However, when postpartum depression is operating the woman has difficulty separating the parenting event from herself and begins to make critical evaluations of herself and/or the infant whenever she is challenged by an infant care task she is unable to handle. The key for differentiating whether the problem lies in lack of skill or insufficient knowledge in task performance versus whether the difficulty reflects depressive symptomatology is through assessment of what the task involves and the frequency of successful outcomes. Women experiencing postpartum depression will experience difficulties with infant care tasks that are considered to be standard for meeting the normal needs of the newborn such as feeding, bathing, grooming and will exhibit low rates of successful outcomes. Another warning sign is that the depressed woman will verbalize with increased frequency that everyday parenting activities are becoming more a source of frustration than satisfying encounters.

Preoccupation or disinterest in the newborn

All mothers express concern about their newborn baby to some degree after childbirth and such anxieties can serve as a healthy stimulus towards good parenting. However, healthy mothers are able to respond favorably when counsel and guidance are offered in attempts to differentiate concerns that are reality based versus those that are exaggerated or fantasied. The depressed postpartum woman may have difficulty differentiating between reality and fantasied concerns such that she develops a preoccupation with perceived threats to the baby's safety and/or her own safety as a mother/woman. Two behavioral responses can become manifested; the woman may develop either an over-indulgence, excessively protective behavioral repertoire or exhibit neglectful, disinterested, aloof approaches to the newborn. Should either behavioral pattern manifest, it is a warning sign that the woman needs help to be relieved of her parenting duties so she can redirect her energies toward resolving the postpartum depression.

Cognitive changes and disturbances

Women who are depressed can experience alterations in their cognitive abilities as the depression persists and becomes more severe. Examples of cognitive changes which can occur are inability to attend to details in daily activities, diminished attention span, difficulty in concentration, inability to complete simple hand-eye coordination tasks, reduction in short-term memory, and difficulty organizing household events she normally manages with relative ease. It is important to know the woman's baseline cognitive functions to appreciate the significance of changes occurring in her present cognitive abilities. When the present cognitive abilities respresent a great deviation from normal baseline behaviors then the cognitive disturbances can be cues that depressive symptomatology is interfering with the woman's functioning. Disturbances in cognitive functioning also reflect that the postpartum depression is at least of moderate intensity and has been operating for sometime. During the time when cognitive disturbances are present, the woman should be relieved of decision-making responsibilities so that help can be sought to reduce the emotional tensions she is experiencing.

Generalized fatigue and feeling that 'all is not well'

The emotional tensions experienced and the fact that unresolved psychological stress only sets into motion a vicious cycle that rapidly escalates into crises, leaves the postpartum depressed woman exhausted. Thus her generalized fatigue is not only legitimate but indeed real and not exaggerated! Unfortunately, due to all the disturbances occurring in her physical body as well as her cognitive and affective functioning she is not in the optimal condition to identify the problem and implement strategies to resolve the depression by herself. Therefore, an early warning sign is her feeling and verbalization that 'all is not well' after childbirth. This vague self statement serves the function of cluing the woman and her family to the painful reality that depression may be cycling in her present situation. All is indeed not well and will not get better without therapeutic assistance. Thus, generalized, vague self-statements made by postpartum women should not be taken lightly, ignored or minimized as they frequently represent the closest articulation to how the woman is perceiving her realities.

Somatic disturbances

Women experiencing postpartum depression can have increased disruptions in their daily physical functioning such as difficulties in sleeping, loss of appetite, increased agitation or psychomotor retardation, diminished interest in sexual and recreational activities. Somatic complaints may escalate especially in terms of neurological functions (tremulousness, headaches, sense of tight constriction around forehead), musculo-skeletal actvities (frequently tired, weaker, unable to complete routine household tasks), gastro-intestinal functions (nausea, vomiting, diarrhea, constipation), and cardio-pulmonary ailments (palpitations, shortness of breath, hyperventilation). If the somatic disturbances are not dealt with in a straightforward manner (after assessment rules out the possibility of a physical diagnostic problem) and put into the perspective of a possible postpartum depression phenomenon, there is the danger that a hypochondriacal pattern can develop because postpartum women frequently receive abundant attention for their reports on physical functioning especially from members of the obstetrical health care system. Even the routine 6 weeks postpartum obstetrical examination is mainly a physical check-up event.

Apathy and despondency

As with any other type of depression, apathetic and despondent behaviors communicate the severity of the disorder. Apathy and despondency take over when other healthier behaviors to reach out for help have failed, such as getting angry, irritable, frustrated, and aggressive. It is as if the woman gives up attempts to rectify her emotional distress. Thus, apathetic and despondent behaviors parallel the woman's sense of failure and hopelessness. Any postpartum woman who exhibits apathy, despondency, and does not exhibit favorable responses to efforts from professionals in the obstetrical health care system, should be referred to a mental health specialist for in-depth therapy work.

Careful review of the above clinical manifestations of postpartum depression indicates that the signs and symptoms are insidious in nature, such as the inability to cope, feelings of inadequacy, irritability and frustrations. At times, the symptoms may appear unrelated to childbirth because of their subtlety. One study described a syndrome termed as 'the postpartum masked depression' which was characterized by such vagues signs as: unexplained irritability, unprovoked hostility in interpersonal relationships, deleterious changes in marital, familial relationships, changes in sexual behaviors, change in relationship with children (especially in the direction of withdrawal and neglect), and initiation of extramarital affairs by women previously monogamous (Lesse & Aronson, 1974). Another author (Tod, 1972) found that many of the depressed women in his sample managed to hide their symptoms from members of the obstetrical profession through false personality projections of extreme well-being. Thus, diagnosis of postpartum depression is a difficult process in both the obstetrical and mental health systems. When women are referred to the mental health specialist their postpartum depression typically gets labeled as 'postpartum psychosis' because of the time lapse since the childbirth events. Also the current Diagnostic and Statistical Manual (DSM III) by the American Psychiatric Association (1980) does not contain criteria for postpartum depression but does for postpartum psychosis.

Onset and duration

The onset of symptoms suggestive of postpartum depression can occur any time after childbirth (Lesse & Aronson, 1974; Vandenbergh, 1980). Several authors report an early manifestation, with peak of depressive symptoms occurring between the third and fourth postpartum day (Yalom et al, 1968; Dalton, 1971; Cone, 1972; Bradley, 1976; Manly et al, 1982). Postpartum depression in this early period has been attributed to hormonal causes due to the fact that there is a precipitous drop in maternal hormonal levels, notably estrogen and progesterone, around the third day after childbirth. Other authors report increased frequency of depressive symptomatology weeks later, especially between the third and eighth postpartum weeks (Pitt, 1968; Affonso, 1982). One study emphasized that depressive symptomatology was likely to occur anytime during the entire postpartum year and if remained unresolved could last for years (Lesse & Aronson, 1974). Systematic studies regarding the onset, duration and causal factors for postpartum depression are generally lacking in the current literature. The present emphasis is to continue assessment for depressive symptomatology beyond the initial first week when most women are exposed to a health care professional during confinement for childbirth. Assessment for depressive symptomatology should also occur weeks later when the woman has returned to the realities of her world and can easily become overwhelmed. The sixth postpartum week has been identified as a vulnerable time period necessitating assessment for depression (Pitt, 1968). Affonso (1982) found that depressive cognitions and affect could be operating earlier, beginning during the second postpartum week, manifesting intensely during the third postpartum week, and continuing into the eighth postpartum week. It has been advocated that assessment for postpartum depression continue after the woman's 6 weeks obstetrical examination when health professionals make the assumption that satisfactory psychological adaptation is paralleling the attainment of adequate physiological adjustment following childbirth (Oakley, 1980; Scarf, 1980). Clearly, more studies are needed on the relationships between temporal factors and postpartum depression.

Influencing variables

Several factors have been reported as contributing to disruptions in a woman's psychological adaptation after childbirth, thereby increasing her vulnerability to manifest signs and symptoms which typically gets labeled as the postpartum depression syndrome. These influencing variables are listed below:

1. Any obstetrical complication that affects the woman's state of comfort, ability for self care and ability to resume care of the household and family (Tod, 1972; Morcos et al, 1979; Danforth, 1982).
2. The women's evaluation of events associated with pregnancy and childbirth, especially regarding critical, confused, ambivalent judgements made about self and/or others (Affonso, 1977; Brown & Harris, 1978).
3. Maternal-role conflicts such as anxieties about mothering tasks and personal insecurities regarding management of maternal responsibilities (Gordon et al, 1965; Kaij & Nilsson, 1972).
4. Disruptions in daily activities and resumption of normal interests due to difficulties in sleeping, eating, and escalation of mood swings (Gordon et al, 1965; Cone, 1972; Kaij & Nilsson, 1972).
5. Behavioural excesses or deficits in mother-infant interactions due to preoccupation and anxieties about the baby's safety or condition; interferences in visual, auditory, tactile stimulation with the infant; critical conclusions drawn about the self and/or infant, and lack of satisfaction with normal infant-care tasks (Benedek, 1970; Klaus & Kennell, 1976; Clark & Affonso, 1979).
6. Lack of social supports to aid in resumption of home care tasks, relief from infant care activities, provision for normal social relationships with other adults, or any perceived alterations in marital relationship or relationships with others (Oakley, 1980; Paykel et al, 1980; Scarf, 1980).

7. Difficulty in evaluating the entire childbirth event as a positive meaningful life experience (Rubin, 1961; Affonso, 1977).

8. Inadequate personality structure leading to neurotic behavioral coping styles (Pitt, 1968; Tod, 1972; Kaij & Nilsson, 1972).

WOMEN'S VULNERABILITY TO POSTPARTUM DEPRESSION

A review of the literature reveals a consistent theme in that only two classes of outcomes regarding postpartum depression are reported: women are classified as either depressed or not. Is it possible that there is a group of women who are presently not being identified because they do not fit into the 'either/or' classification system relative to postpartum depression? A study was undertaken to address this question (Affonso, 1982). A cognitive theoretical approach was chosen to develop an assessment method of postpartum depression because the recent literature advocated that cognitive factors were prominent in the development of depression after childbirth (Manly et al, 1982), and that investigation of perceived consequences of events was a productive area of research regarding depressive cognitions (Gong-Guy & Hammer, 1980). 80 women participated in the study by completing a total of five questionnaires via a self-report, return by mail survey, conducted during the third and eighth postpartum weeks. The purpose of the study was to assess if there was a relationship between postpartum adaptation and a woman's vulnerability to postpartum depression. The third postpartum week was chosen because it represented a time period when women were settled into some type of home routine reflecting a level of postpartum adaptation which could then be assessed. The third postpartum week also permitted differentiation of symptomatology attributed to the blues syndrome versus that of depression. The eighth postpartum week was also chosen for reassessment because the realities of the woman's world would be fully operating by then. Also any perceived consequences from the woman's daily events which had been converted into depressive cognitions could be assessed adequately by this time period. Postpartum adaptation was assessed by a newly developed 35-item instrument, known as the Inventory of Postpartum Adaptation (IPA), which focused on five selected areas of adaptation. The five areas were:

1. Disturbances in activities of daily living as measured by sleep, eating, moods, sexual patterns, level of energy, ability to care

for self, baby, and household

2. Labor-delivery events as measured by preoccupation with the experience, self-evaluation of how the events were handled, overall evaluation of the childbirth experience, presence of any disappointments, sadness or anger

3. Interactions with the new baby as measured by degree of comfort when with the baby, pleasures while caring for the infant, presence of any negative and positive emotions when with the baby, thoughts of 'something bad happening to the baby,' confused feelings or thoughts about the baby, any angry feelings toward the baby, and perceived comfort at being a mother

4. Social supports network as measured by relationship with infant's father, ability for fun activities with the family, degree of social activities with other adults, perception of emotional support received from family, and any sense of isolation from other adults

5. Self construal system as measured by the woman's rating on the 'goodness' of herself, how she manages her many roles, perception of her physical attractiveness, predominant mood after childbirth, outlook for her future, acknowledgement of any depressive feelings present, and any thoughts of suicide.

The presence of any psychological discomforts in the woman's postpartum adaptation during the third week was assessed by the Psychological Screening Inventory (Lanyon, 1973) which is a 130 items self-administered, true or false instrument used to identify individuals experiencing emotional discomforts due to sense of alienation, non-conformity behaviors, or increased anxiety leading to somatic symptomatology and neurotic coping styles. The presence of depressive symptomatology during the eighth postpartum week was assessed by two instruments. The Beck Depressive Inventory (Beck, 1967) is a 21 item, self-rating instrument based on a cognitive theory of depression and measures the presence and severity of depressive symptomatology in general. The second instrument is known as Pitt's Questionnaire (Pitt, 1968) which is a 24 item, answered 'yes,' 'no,' 'I don't know' instrument designed to assess 12 factors specific to the depression following childbirth such as sleep, inability to relax, sense of attractiveness, appetite, sexual interest, concerns about the baby, ability to remember details, confidence in self as a woman and mother.

The findings from this preliminary study indicate that there is a significant relationship between selected aspects of a woman's postpartum adaptation and her vulnerability to depression. These selected, significant areas are:

instability in moods
difficulties in maintaining an adequate eating schedule for one's self
diminished energy level
negative emotions while with the baby
lack of comfort in being a mother
difficulties in relationship with baby's father
lack of time for fun activities
diminished opportunity for social activities
perception of insufficient emotional support from family
sense of isolation from other adults
not feeling good about one's self
difficulties in management of roles as mother, wife, resumption of career
perception of being physically unattractive
presence of depression feelings
dim outlook of the future
presence of suicidal ideation.

Such findings support the cognitive framework that depression is related to critical interpretations and judgements made about the self and events in one's world rather than merely consequences from the events per se (Beck, 1967). The findings also demonstrate that the phenomenon known as postpartum depression is related to events in a woman's life that influence selected critical areas of functioning, specifically her moods, essential day to day activities, especially regarding eating and energy level, comfort in the mothering role, social supports available, and the cognitions by which she evaluates herself as someone of value and worth. The study also supports the literature that revealed that approximately 3–6% of women experience depression following childbirth (Pitt, 1968; Tod, 1972). However, the results also brought attention to a new group of women who could be classified as experiencing difficulties in their postpartum adaptation and may be vulnerable to depression. The results indicated 10% of the sample could be classified as vulnerable to postpartum depression, demonstrating there does exist a group of women who are presently not identified as needing help in their postpartum adaptation when only the 'either/or' classification is used by professionals in the obstetrical/mental health care systems. What are the consequences regarding mental health functioning to post-partum women who are vulnerable to depression? The answer to this question can only be speculated at this time since the concept of vulnerability remains undefined and is yet to be researched in the current postpartum literature.

There are several other findings from the study worthy of mention in terms of enhancing an understanding of postpartum depression and identifying future directions for research on the topic. These findings are summarized below.

1. Of particular interest were the four areas of daily functioning in a woman's life that changed significantly after the arrival of the baby. These areas were sleep patterns, eating schedule, moods, and energy level; all changed toward the less favorable direction of adjustment. Thus, these four areas are worthy of investigation for better understanding of postpartum adaptation and a woman's vulnerability to depressive symptomatology.

2. The majority of women reported increased preoccupation with the events that surround childbirth and most women indicated such thoughts were of a positive nature. However, 30% of the sample reported ambivalent feelings (especially confusion) about the events that occurred in their lives. Thus, further assessment on the theme of ambivalence regarding a women's frequent thinking about her childbirth experience is worthy of additional investigation, especially the exploration of any relationship between ambivalent thoughts and postpartum depression.

3. The assessment on mother-infant interactions revealed more than 50% of the sample reported experiencing uncomfortable emotions such as fear, tension, confusion while with the new baby during both the third and eighth week; 55–64% reported thoughts of 'something bad' happening to the new baby; 25–35% reported ambivalent feelings while performing infant care activities and discomforts at being a mother with increased changes toward being more uncomfortable by the eighth postpartum week. Thus, the area of how a woman is perceiving the events involved in early parenting, the judgements made about herself as a mother, and evaluations of how she perceives the infant is feeling towards her as a mother are all worthy of further investigation. For so long the emphasis in the postpartum period has been on how the infant is responding to parenting that there has not been enough attention on the cognitive-affective evaluations of parents about their own parenting experiences.

4. Assessment of a postpartum woman's social support system indicated that the majority of women sampled had insufficient social supports in terms of diminished opportunities for fun activities, difficulties with resumption back into the adult social world, and perceptions of inadequate emotional support from family and friends. Such a finding supports the social perspective on depression which advocates that the social structure surrounding the childbearing experience can contribute to postpartum depression (Oakley, 1980; Scarf, 1980).

5. Finally, assessment of a woman's self construal system indicated all questions on postpartal adaptation in this area were found to be significantly correlated with vulnerability to postpartum depression. Such a finding supports those authors who have speculated that cognitive factors contribute to postpartum depression (Manly et al, 1982). Thus, for future directions it is just as important to assess the evaluations a woman makes about herself and her future after childbirth, as it is to evaluate her competency in performing infant care tasks and resumption of household and family responsibilities. Specifically, further studies are needed on factors that influence how a woman is able to maintain stability in her moods, her perceptions of being ugly versus attractive, her evaluations of how she is managing her multiple roles, and what types of data she uses to evaluate the goodness of herself. Of special interest, all women sampled in this study reported experiencing feelings of depression at least some of the time during both the third and eighth postpartum week.

NURSING ASSESSMENT

Assessment is prerequisite to intervention, and yet identification of women who are vulnerable to depression continues to be excluded as a standard goal of the nursing care plans developed for postpartum women. Assessment for postpartum depression involves a twofold process:

1. Differentiation of whether the clinical phenonmenon the woman presents is a 'postpartum blues' reaction versus a postpartum depression
2. Casefindings for early signs suggestive of depression following childbirth.

Postpartum blues vs postpartum depression

It is not unusual to witness a postpartum woman experiencing

transitory states of emotional distress and feelings of sadness. Therefore, it is important to differentiate between a blues reaction versus a
depressive reaction in postpartum women. A syndrome referred to
as 'postpartum blues' has been described in the literature as a
mild-subclinical depressive response in relation to selected environmental variables (Liakos et al 1972). Postpartum blues has also been
referred to as a 'hypersensitive emotional state' resulting in frequent
mood disturbances rather than being a depressive syndrome (Derbolowsky et al, 1979). The postpartal blues reaction is characterized
by symptoms listed in Table 8.2. There are several criteria that
differentiate the hypersensitive emotional state known as postpartum blues from the clinically significant syndrome of postpartum
depression. The main criteria are related to the (a) severity and
persistence of the depressive reaction, (b) its effects on the woman's
daily functioning, and (c) the types of behavioral manifestations.
Reactions indicative of postpartum blues are largely transitory in
nature and although the emotional distress is viewed as intense by
the woman, the 'blues episode' frequently does not persist beyond
one week's duration when mood stability can be observed. The
course of postpartum depression, however, will usually continue for
weeks and/or months with the woman not making progress in cognitive-affective functioning as postpartum weeks accrue. Another
criteria is that a woman experiencing postpartum blues may be

Table 8.2 Manifestations of 'postpartum blues' reaction

---

1. Early manifestation in the puerperium, between the second to seventh day (first postpartum week)
2. Short duration, with symptoms lasting on average from 2–7 days
3. Highly reactive to stimuli in the external environment especially in terms of absence of supportive person, economic constraints, unwanted pregnancy, undesired sex of infant, inadequacy of living conditions, interruptions in career goals
4. Mood swings can be stabilized by environmental manipulations in a short period of time, although frequency in mood alterations can continue to occur at different periods of time in reactions to an external event
5. Statements made by the woman tend to be critical of external, environmental variables rather than be directed to the internal, psychological self. (i.e. blaming lack of money for an inadequate meal versus blaming of self)
6. Daily activities such as eating, sleeping, care of baby, self, and household may be difficult at times but she is able to manage daily routines with or without transient sources of help
7. Frequent crying and tearfulness are prominent behavioral manifestations. Crying episodes may be preceded and/or followed by verbal communications of emotional distress which serve two functions: (a) allow the woman to express her needs and (b) facilitate her active seeking of help effectively from the environment. Crying episodes are largely reactive to environmental stimuli

---

emotionally stressed but can continue to perform activities of daily living with occasional help. The woman basically can maintain control over care of herself, the new baby, and household-social affairs. However, a woman experiencing postpartum depression will have increasing difficulties with day to day function in such essential parameters as sleep, eating, parenting, sex, and recreation. The mood swings can be replaced by apathy and despondency if the depression persists. The depressed woman is in a vulnerable situation because she will not be able to manage without assistance. Help is necessary for working through both the physical responsibilities as well as the mental-emotional distress. The third criterion category involves the behavioral manifestations. Women with postpartum blues will exhibit more emotional hypersensitivity especially in terms of mood instability, be prone to hystrionic type behaviors, and be highly reactive to the environment especially regarding events related to childbearing such as occurrences during the labor-delivery and parenting encounters. Such behaviors are frequently manifested early in the postpartum period and are time limited; symptoms peak around the third to fourth postpartum day and frequently do not last beyond the second to early part of the third postpartum week. However, depressed postpartum women will exhibit more process-type behaviors which are insidious and vague in nature. Initially, the woman is able to express verbally the feeling that 'something is wrong' and communicates this to her environment by pleas for help through some reactive type of behaviors such as anger, frustrations, mood swings. However as the depression remains unresolved into weeks and/or months, the nature of her symptomatology changes character toward more process oriented psychopathology in which mood swings convert into apathy and despondency, anger turns into hostility, and aggression is replaced by withdrawal. Table 8.3 provides a differential diagnosis of these two reactions.

It is important to differentiate between postpartum blues and postpartum depression because each dictates a different plan for intervention. The former will respond favorably to supportive mea-

Table 8.3 Differential diagnosis of postpartum blues versus postpartum depression

Criteria	Postpartum blues	Postpartum depression
Severity and persistence	A. Transitory symptoms disappear with time	A. Process orientation symptoms become more complex, convert to other symptoms with time

	B. Frequently manifest in 1st postpartum week, does not persist for many weeks	B. Persist beyond 1st postpartum week
Effects on day to day function	A. Care of self, baby, household may be disrupted, but woman is able to function adequately B. Generally is able to manage with or without temporary help C. Patterns of eating, sleeping, moods, socializations may be disturbed but *return to baseline* levels occurs with time D. Feelings of tiredness occur but energy is replenished by periods of rest and relaxation and the woman is able to continue daily routines	A. Deterioration in ability to care for self, baby, household as postpartum days progress B. Unable to manage over time even when temporary help is provided C. As time progresses, disturbances in eating, sleeping, moods, socializations become more severe, such that the woman's *baseline converts* is a negative direction D. Generalized fatigue permeates such that day to day routines cannot continue. Attempts at rest and sleep do not make women feel more energetic, and complaints of 'feeling more tired' increase over time
Types of behavioral manifestations	A. Woman highly reactive to environmental stimuli relative to childbearing events B. Reactive behaviors common, as frequently seen with crying, increased verbalizations. Responses have a hysterical style C. Effectively can communicate with others annd elicit supportive help from the environment D. Mood disturbances escalate but stabilizes with time.	A. Symptoms are unprovoked and may appear unrelated to childbearing. Woman is less reactive to her environment B. Process behaviors common as manifested by more subtle vague responses which appear perplexing to the woman and those around her C. Communication skills is reduced in effectiveness and pleas for help take on an aggressive/hostile style D. Mood disturbances persist and convert to apathy and despondency over time.

sures, environmental manipulations, and involve short-term strategies, while the latter will dictate relief from parenting and involve a long-term course of structured therapy for reversal of symptomatology to protect the woman's mental health functioning.

Early casefinding

Early casefinding for the potential problem of depression following childbirth involve the following crucial assessment areas:

Predominant moods

Although mood swings are largely anticipated as part of a woman's recovery from childbirth, a re-education regarding the significance of mood instability is necessary for childbearing women, their families, as well as obstetrical health professionals. Persistence of mood disturbance beyond 5–7 days duration should not be taken lightly, especially if episodes of mood swings become more frequent as postpartum days progress. Of special significance are mood alterations that occur without precipitating events and such unprovoked moodiness persists beyond the first postpartum month. A crucial assessment technique is to ask the woman and her family to describe her predominant mood since the birth of her baby, as they are the experts as to what her baseline is regarding mood behavior.

Daily functioning

Day to day functioning is a good indicator of how well the woman's personality structure has incorporated the recent events surrounding pregnancy and childbirth. Thus, difficulties in managing the routine interest in daily activities are early indicators of psychological post-partum maladaptation. Assessment includes how the woman manages a triad of events — herself, the new baby, and household/family affairs. Frequently, assessment emphasizes how well she is handling parenting and household tasks. However, of more significance is how well she is able to manage herself such that her day to day functioning is not disturbed, or that her baseline functioning after childbirth has realigned to another level of optimal coping. A recent study demonstrated the assessment of eating and sleeping be-haviours is an important indicator of postpartum psychological adaptation (Affonso, 1982).

Most women will have altered sleep patterns during the first 3–4 weeks after childbirth until the newborn establishes longer intervals between sleep and wakefulness states. Therefore, persistence of disturbed sleep patterns after the first postpartum month serves as a warning sign for the potential of depressive symptomatology. An earlier sign of possible depression is alterations in eating schedule beyond the second postpartum week, especially regarding missed meals, diminished appetite, or deficiencies in nutritional intake. The combination of disturbed eating and sleeping patterns is a predictor that energy levels will rapidly diminish, such that generalized fatigue permeates the new altered baseline level of daily functioning.

Evaluations of self as a parent

Nurses have typically focused on helping women make the transitions to mothering by teaching the 'how to's' of infant care. It is considered standard practice in many hospital obstetrical services for postpartum women to be exposed to some type of parenting classes conducted frequently by nurses. However, this teaching-learning modality is no longer sufficient and certainly antiquated if professionals assume that learning occurs simply because content is provided. It is important to go one step forward and assess the evaluations women make about themselves as consequences to their early parenting encounters. Critical assessment data useful in casefinding women vulnerable to postpartum depression can be obtained by asking women to evaluate their comfort at being a mother and what are their *affective* responses during their mothering encounters. Another useful assessment strategy is to ask the woman what she perceives are her *baby's feelings* toward her as a mother.

Social supports

There is appreciation that supportive actions by significant persons are crucial to the emotional adjustment of a woman following childbirth. However, it is also important to assess the woman's perceptions of her progression back into the social adult world. Too often postpartum women are burdened by infant and household tasks that they sacrifice adult socializations because these are construed to be of least importance amidst the many priorities in the parenting situations. However, there is strong evidence to indicate that diminished socializations contribute to depressive symptomatology (Coyne, 1976; Oakley, 1980). Thus, it is just as important to ask a woman about her socializations with other adults as it is to assess if she interacts with her new baby. Diminished social contacts with other adults can escalate emotional and social withdrawal which is a precursor to depressive cognitions about one's self.

Self-constructs

Finally, it is just as important to assess the types of evaluations and judgements a woman makes about herself following childbirth, as it is to assess if she is bleeding or having an infection. As bleeding and infection are of danger to her physical recovery and health, so are negative, critical self constructs (thought process) of danger to ber emotional and mental health. A recent study (Affonso, 1982) provided examples of important assessment areas, such as rating the goodness of one's self, degree of physical attractiveness perceived, judgements about how well one is managing multiple roles, and outlook for one's future. To date, assessment of such variables have yet to be integrated into the 6 weeks postpartum check up which is the final interface for the postpartum woman until another conception occurs or complications ensue.

Therapeutic strategies

It is important to appreciate that postpartum depression is a phenomenon likely to be fully operating when the childbearing woman has exited out of the obstetrical health care system via the 6 weeks postpartum check-up. Therefore, a primary prevention approach which employs cognitive therapeutic strategies is predicted to have optimum benefits in dealing with the problem of depressive symptomatology during the postpartum period. The period following childbirth when depression is likely to originate and behaviourally manifest is considered to be the entire first postpartum year (Lesse & Aronson, 1974). However, the specific time period when a woman is especially susceptible to depressive symptomatology is currently unknown. Several recent studies have indicated the first, third, sixth and eighth postpartum weeks to be vulnerable time periods (Pitt, 1968; Affonso, 1982; Manly et al, 1982). Thus, it can be predicted that most postpartum woman who experience depression will be in environments that have little proximity to health professionals and therefore any attempts to prevent the problem by casefinding women who are especially vulnerable to depression can be considered a therapeutic strategy.

A primary goal of employing cognitive therapy for dealing with depressed individuals is to work through the person's thought processes in the hopes of preventing, altering or reversing any critical, negative cognitions the person is developing by which they evaluate themselves, the world, and the future (Beck, 1967). Negative cognitions are believed to result from disturbances in logical thinking styles as manifested by four types of errors which can lead to depressive symptomatology. These are : (1) error of arbitrary interference in which conclusions are drawn in the absence of insufficient data; (2) error of selective abstraction in which conclusions are based on consideration of only one of the many elements involved in a situations; (3) error of overgeneralization in which an overall conclusion is made on the basis of evaluation on only a single event; (4) error of magnification or minimization in which gross errors in judgement of one's performance are made due to maximizing failures or minimizing successes (Beck, 1967).

These four forms of errors are not mutually exclusive thus, a vicious cycle is nurtured once the process of error is operating in the individual's cognitive style of dealing with the world. The postpartum woman is especially vulnerable to errors in her logical thinking due to the complexity of events she must cope with once childbirth is completed. Consider the following examples of the many cognitve errors frequently made by postpartum women even during the short hospital stay of approximately only 3 days after delivery:

Conclusion that something is wrong with the infant or self because the scheduled visiting time with the baby has been altered (arbitrary interference error)

Conclusion that your baby does not like you or that you are not an adequate mother because the baby ate more when fed by the nurse (selection abstraction error)

Conclusion that the woman failed in the childbirth event because the desired sex infant was not produced (error in overgeneralization)

Decision made to have minimal contact with the infant because of conclusions that one is not a good mother due to difficulties in diapering, bathing, and/or consoling fussy behaviors (error in magnification of failures or minimizations of successes).

The above are only four examples of an endless list frequently heard by nurses working with postpartum women. Examples of suggested cognitive therapeutic strategies for reversing or minimizing such negative cognitions in postpartum women are as follows:

Listen carefully to the woman's self reported statements which reflect that some type of evaluation, judgement, or conclusion has been made and help her to reasses the data such that a different, less critical, more neutral conclusion can be arrived at.

Help the woman to gain some degree of neutrality in her cognitions and decision-making process by guiding and counseling her to keep events that occur in her environment separate from her cognitive-affective responses. Attempts to depersonalize selected aspects of the childbirth events which are beyond her control will help the woman to maintain a reality-based perspective. The reality perspective can then become the foundation upon which she integrates the many childbirth events into a meaningful life experience.

Assist the woman to expand her options for choosing alternatives as to the types of evaluations, judgements, conclusions she will make. Alternatives are expanded when data collection is enhanced and degrees of freedom to make choices are perceived when the data base is rich and reality-based. Nurses are tremendous resources by which postpartum women can find missing data, clarify information that is confusing, and get help in selecting which data is to be used or eliminated in the process of drawing logical conclusions. Working with the data involves a process referred to as 'cognitive mapping' which supplies the energy source for the woman's future affective and behavioral functioning as consequence from the childbearing life experience.

Finally, nurses can help postpartum women to plan and organize the means by which they can return back into the social adult world. Nurses are presently assisting postpartum women in learning how to monitor their fundus, check for infection and other complications, prepare for making choices regarding family planning techniques, and develop skills and competencies in early parenting. There is now evidence indicating good social skills are an important protective shield against postpartum depression (Oakley, 1980; Affonso, 1982). Thus, nurses can reinforce attempts made by women for social contacts such as telephone conversations, visitors, early discharge, and reinforce the notion that relief time from parenting via babysitters is as important as feeding the baby or checking one's lochia flow. Too often, societal myths generate guilt feelings when women express desire to be relieved of their mothering responsibilities and such myths promote distortions in the stereotype of what is a 'good mother'. Nurses can be instrumental in advocating that attention to the self and activation of adult socializations are indeed good mental health strategies in promoting postpartum psychological adaptation.

The above are only examples of the types of cognitive therapeutic strategies that can be employed for preventing and/or minimizing the incidence of postpartum depression. As the phenomenon of depression in postpartum women is only beginning to be understood in terms of theory development, the identification of strategies for assessing and dealing with the problem poses a future challenge to the nursing profession.

REFERENCES

Affonso D 1977 Missing pieces — A study of postpartum feelings. Birth and Family Journal 4(4): 159–165
Affonso D 1982 Assessment of women's postpartal adaptation as indicator of vulnerability to depression. Unpublished dissertation. University of Arizona, Department of Psychology. Tucson, Arizona
American Psychiatric Association 1980 Diagnostic and statistical manual of mental disorders, 3rd edn. APA, Washington, D. C.
Arkowitz H 1980 Depressive symptomatology. Unpublished manuscript. University of Arizona. Department of Psychology, Tucson, Arizona
Bardon D 1972 Puerperal depression. Psychosomatic Medicine to Obstetrics and Gynecology, 3rd International Congress, Karger: Basel, p 335–337
Beck A 1967 Depression: Clinical, experimental and theoretical aspects. Hoeber, New York
Benedek T 1970 Motherhood and nurturing. In: Anthony E, Benedek T (eds). Parenthood: Its psychology and psychopathology. Little Brown, Boston
Bradley C 1976 The effects of hospital experience on postpartum feelings and attitudes of women. Unpublished doctoral dissertation. University of British Columbia, Canada
Brown G, Harris T 1978 Social origins of depression: A study of psychiatric disorder in women. Tavistock Publications, London
Cameron N 1963 Personality development and psychopathology, a dynamic approach. Houghton Mifflin, Boston
Caplan G 1959 Concepts of mental health and consultation. U.S. Department of Health, Education and Welfare, Children's Bureau, Washington, D.C.
Clark A, Affonso D 1979 Childbearing: A nursing perspective, 2nd edn. F.A. Davis Publishers, Philadelphia
Clarke M, Williams A 1979 Depression in women after perinatal death. Lancet 8122: 916–917
Cone B 1972 Puerperal depression. Psychosomatic Medicine in Obstetrics and Gynecology, 3rd International Congress, Karger: Basel, p 355–357
Coyne J 1976 Depression and the response of others. Journal of Abnormal Psychology 85: 186–193
Dalton K 1971 Prospective study into puerperal depression. British Journal of Psychology 118: 689–692
Danforth D 1982 Textbook of obstetrics and gynecology, 4th edn. Harper and Row, New York
Derbolowsky J, Benkert O, Ott L, Laakmann G, Weissenbacher E, Von Zerssen D 1979 The postpartum blues — A depressive syndrome. In: Carenza L, Zichella L (eds) Emotion and reproduction, 5th International Congress of Psychosomatic Obstetrics and Gynecology, Academic Press, New York 823–829, 1979
Deutsch H 1944/5 The psychology of women. Grune & Stratton, New York vol. I (1944), vol. II (1945)

Freud S 1957 Mourning and melancholia (1917). Collected papers, vol. 4 Hogarth
    Press, London
Gallant D, Simpson E (eds) 1976 Depression: Behavioral, biochemical, diagnostic and
    treatment concepts. Wiley, New York
Gelder M 1978 Hormones and postpartum depression. In: Sandler M (ed), Mental
    illness in pregnancy and the puerperium. Oxford University Press, Oxford
Gong-Guy E, Hammen C 1980 Causal perceptions of stressful events in depressed and
    nondepressed outpatients. Journal of Abnormal Psychology 89: 662–669
Gordon R, Kapostins E, Gordon K 1965 Factors in postpartum emotional
    adjustment. Obstetrics and Gynecology 25: 158–166
Hamilton J 1962 Postpartum psychiatric problems. Mosby, St Louis
Kaij L, Nilsson A 1972 Emotional and psychotic illness following childbirth. In:
    Howell J (ed), Modern perspectives in psycho-obstetrics. Brunner/Mazel, New
    York
Kane F 1968 Emotional and cognitive disturbances in early puerperium. British
    Journal of Psychiatry 114: 99–102
Klaus M, Kennell J 1976 Maternal-infant bonding Mosby, St Louis
Kubler-Ross E 1969 On death and dying. MacMillan, New York
Lanyon R 1973 Psychological screening inventory. Research Psychologists Press,
    New York
LeMasters E 1965 Parenthood as a crisis. In: Parad H (ed) Crisis intervention:
    Selected readings. Family Service Association of America, New York
Lesse S, Aronson L 1974 Masked depression. Jason Aronson, New York p 102–103
Lewinsohn P 1975 The behavioral study and treatment of depression. In: Hersen M
    (ed), Progress in Behavior Modification vol. 1. Academic Press, New York
Liakos A, Panayotakopoulous K, Lyketsos G, Kaskarelis D 1972 Depressive and
    neurotic symptoms in the puerperium. Psychosomatic medicine in obstetrics and
    gynecology, 3rd International Congress. Karger, Basel, p 343–346
Manly P, McMahon R, Bardley C, Davidson P 1982 Depressive attributional style
    and depression following childbirth. Journal of Abnormal Psychology 91(4):
    245–254
Mercer R 1981 The nurse and maternal tasks of early postpartum. American Journal
    of Maternal Child Nursing 6 (5): 341–346, Sept.–Oct.
Morcos F, Funke-Ferber J 1979 Anxiety and depression in the mother and father and
    their relationship to physical complications of pregnancy and labour. In: Carenza
    L, Zichella L (eds), Emotion and reproduction 5th International Congress of
    Psychosomatic Obstetrics and Gynecology, Academic Press, New York p 757–765
Oakley A 1980 Women confined: Toward a sociology of childbirth. Oxford
    University Press, Oxford
Paykel E, Emms E, Fletcher J, Rassaby E 1980 Life events and social support in
    puerperal depression. British Journal of Psychiatry 136: 339–346
Pitt B 1968 A typical depression following childbirth. British Journal of Psychiatry
    114: 1325–1335
Pritchard J, MacDonald P 1980 William's obstetrics, 16th edn. Appleton-Century
    Crofts, New York
Rehm L 1976 Assessment of depression. In: Hersen M, Bellack A (eds), Behavioral
    assessment: A practical handbook. Pergamon Press, Oxford
Rubin R 1961 Basic maternal behavior. Nursing Outlook November: 638–687
Seligman M 1975 Helplessness: On depression, development and health. W. H.
    Freeman, San Francisco
Scarf M 1980 Unfinished business: Pressure point in the lives of women. Doubleday,
    New York
Steiner M 1979 Psychobiology of mental disorders associated with childbearing: An
    overview. Acta Psychiatrica Scandinavica 60: 449–464
Teuting P, Koslow S, Hirschfeld R 1981 Special report on depression. Rockville,

MD: National Institute of Mental Health

Tod E 1972 Puerperal depression. Psychosomatic medicine in obstetrics and gynecology, 3rd International Congress, Karger, Basel, p 338–340

Vandenbergh R 1980 Postpartum depression. Clinical Obstetrics and Gynecology 23: 1105–1111

Yalom I, Lunde D, Moos R, Hamburg D 1968 Postpartum blues syndrome: a description and related variables. Archives of General Psychiatry 18: 16–20

PART TWO

Bibliography

Psychosocial aspects of prenatal care

Program planning of nursing care and nursing services for prenatal clients is heavily influenced by changing consumer demand. The services now expected by the couple in their prenatal care include not only traditional medical supervision but also health teaching with a disease prevention/health promotion/self care philosophy. It is the nurse, in many cases, who is the health professional with the greatest and closest contact with prenatal clients, in a health teaching role. She is therefore in perhaps the best position to evaluate the effectiveness of existing prenatal programs, and to make recommendations for program modifications. Increasingly, the presence and influence of significant others in the pregnant woman's life — husband, extended family, friends, resource people — are considered when supportive/educative/compensatory nursing care is provided to the client. It is recognized that the woman is not alone in experiencing changes in self perception during the pregnancy period. The husband, and significant others who anticipate continued close involvement with the family, also experience a period of re-evaluation of their roles and consideration of their strengths and weaknesses. It is also recognized that the pregnant woman's perception of a reliable support system in her life has a direct relationship with both a positive pregnancy experience and positive pregnancy outcome. In fact, the 'client' becomes the pregnant woman and her support group, the term 'family centred nursing care' indicating this change in nursing orientation. As well as considering the multidimensional physical and psychosocial changes experienced in pregnancy by the couple, the psychosocial changes experienced internally, by the mother alone, deserve some consideration. Even when a reliable support system exists and the pregnant woman can refer to significant others in order to acknowledge the reality of her pregnancy and its impact on her, both in the present and the future, there remain some psychological processes which remain uniquely hers. These internal tasks benefit in an indirect way from prenatal services — particularly supportive activities. Anxiety, a manifestation of coping with crisis and therefore present during pregnancy, has been discussed by numerous authors using a variety of variables. Significant relationships have been shown to be present by many authors. Recognizing the effects that maternal anxiety may have on pregnancy outcome, it becomes a topic deserving some deliberation when considering the aims, objectives and design of prenatal programs. The term 'vulnerability' is used to describe a sense of susceptibility, of weakness, and implies a need for protection. It has been used by a few authors to describe a feeling which they state occurs in the pregnant woman by virtue of pregnancy being a crisis period. There seem, then, to be implications in nursing practice, for the fostering of a climate perceived as 'safe' where supportive and therapeutic exchanges may take place.

Astbury J 1980 The crisis of childbirth: Can information and childbirth education help? Journal of Psychosomatic Research 24: 9–14

Ball J A 1981 Effects of present patterns of maternity care on the emotional needs of mothers. Parts 1 and 2. Midwives Chronicle 94: 151–154; 94: 198–202

Beebe Thompson J 1981 Nurse midwives and health promotion during pregnancy. Original Article Series, March of Dimes XVII 6: 29–57

Benedek T 1949 The psychosomatic implications of the primary unit: Mother child. American Journal of Orthopsychiatry 19: 642–654

Bibring G L, Valenstein A F 1959 Psychoanalytic aspects of pregnancy. Psychoanalytic Study of the Child 14: 113–119

Bibring G L 1961 A study of the psychological processes in pregnancy of the earliest mother-child relationship. Psychoanalytic Study of the Child 16: 9–23

Caplan G 1957 Psychological aspects of maternity care. American Journal of Public Health 47: 25–31

Carey J 1981 First trimester prenatal counselling in private practice. Journal of Obstetrics Gynecology and Neonatal Nursing 10: 336–339

Carlson B 1978 Using 'body image' findings in nursing care. American Journal of Orthopsychiatry 39: 788–797

Colman A D, Colman L L 1973 Pregnancy as an altered state of consciousness. Birth and the Family Journal 1: 7–11

Davids A 1961 Psychological Study of emotional factors in pregnancy. A preliminary report. Psychosomatic Medicine 23:

Davids A 1961 Anxiety pregnancy and childbirth abnormalities. Psychosomatic Medicine 23: 74–77

Dodge J A 1981 Prenatal events and subsequent developments. American Journal of Maternal and Child Health 6: 242, 246, 248

Fawcett J 1978 Body image and the pregnant couple. American Journal of Maternal Child Nursing 3: 227–233

Ferguson I 1977 A psychological approach to pregnancy and childbirth: some aspects which should concern midwives. Midwives Chronicle 90: 187–188

Field P A 1982 What this country needs now... nurses prepared to work with today's parents to revolutionize family-newborn care. The Canadian Nurse: 37–40

Glazer G 1980 Anxiety levels and concerns among pregnant women. Research in

Nursing and Health 3: 107–113

Griffith S 1976 Pregnancy as an event with crisis potential for marital partners: a study of interpersonal needs. Journal of Obstetrics Gynecology and Neonatal Nursing 5: 35–38

Hrobsley D M 1977 Transition to parenthood: a balancing of needs. Nursing Clinics of North America 12: 457–468

Jarraki-Zadeh A 1969 Emotional and cognitive changes in pregnancy and early puerperium. British Journal of Psychiatry 115: 797–805

Kitzinger S 1977 Anxiety in pregnancy. American Journal of Maternal and Child Health 2: 358–360

Kleinman C 1977 Psychological processes during pregnancy. Perspectives in Psychiatric Care XV: 175–178

Lee G 1982 Relationship of self concept during late pregnancy to neonatal perception. Journal of Obstetrics Gynecology and Neonatal Nursing 11: 186–190

Leijer M 1977 Psychological changes accompanying pregnancy and motherhood. Genetic Psychology Monographs 95: 55–96

Lerner B 1967 On the need to be pregnant. International Journal Psychological Analysis 48: 288–296

Parks J 1951 Emotional reactions to pregnancy. American Journal of Obstetrics and Gynecology 62: 339–345

Petersen Tilden V 1980 A developmental conceptual framework for the maturational crisis of pregnancy. Western Journal of Nursing Research 2: 667–685

Rich C 1979 A multigravida's work at organization during pregnancy. Maternal Child Nursing Journal 8: 195–206

Rich O J 1978 The sociogram: a tool for depicting support in pregnancy. Maternal Child Nursing Journal 7: 1–10

Richardson P 1981 Woman's perceptions of their dyadic relationships during pregnancy. Maternal Child Nursing Journal 10: 159–176

Richardson P 1982 Significant relationships and their impact on childbearing: a review. Maternal Child Nursing Journal 11: 17–40

Rubin R 1970 Cognitive style in pregnancy. American Journal of Nursing 70: 502–508

Rubin R 1975 Maternal tasks in pregnancy. Maternal Child Nursing Journal 4: 143–153

Sticher J F, Bowden M S, Reimer E D 1978 Pregnancy: a shared emotional experience. Maternal Child Nursing Journal 3: 153–157

Swaffield L 1982 What about mother? Nursing Times 78: 93–94

Tannes L 1969 Developmental tasks in pregnancy. In Bergesar B (ed) Current Concepts in Clinical Nursing. Mosby, St Louis, p 292–297

Tippling V G 1981 The vulnerability of a primipara during the antepartal period. Maternal Child Nursing Journal 10: 61–77

Tulman L J 1981 Theories of maternal attachment. Advances in Nursing Science 3: 7–14

Van Muiswinkel J 1974 Vulnerability expressed by a primigravida. Maternal Child Nursing Journal 3: 219–234

Waleko K F 1974 Manifestations of a multigravida's feelings of vulnerability. Maternal Child Nursing Journal 3: 103–131

Maternal attachment and bonding

Countless articles on bonding and maternal fetal attachment have been published in the last decade. Public pressure is being placed on institutions and personnel involved in the provision of maternity care to promote measures which encourage bonding. The authors presented in this section were selected as representative of a variety of theoretical viewpoints related to maternal-fetal attachment. Theories of attachment; long-term effects of maternal-newborn separation; bonding in traditional settings vis-à-vis birthing centers; effects of illness on bonding; and the relationship of attachment to abuse are some of the concerns explored by the authors. The literature will provide a useful overview for those interested in further exploration of this topic.

Ainsworth M D 1979 Infant-mother attachment. American Psychologist 34: 932–937
Ali Z, Lowry M 1981 Early maternal-child contact: effects on later behaviour. Development Medicine Child Neurology 23: 337–345
Atkins R N 1981 Finding one's father: the mother's contribution to early father representations. Journal of American Academic Psychoanalysis 9: 539–559
Avant K 1979 Nursing diagnosis: maternal attachment. Advances in Nursing Science 2: 45–55
Avant K C 1981 Anxiety as a potential factor affecting maternal attachment. Journal of Obstetrics Gynecology and Neonatal Nursing 10: 416–419
Berger L R 1980 Parental guilt: self-induced and iatrogenic. Clinical Pediatrics (Saunders, Philadelphia) 19: 499–500
Boudreaux M 1981 Maternal attachment of high-risk mothers with well newborns: a pilot study. Journal of Obstetrics Gynecology and Neonatal Nursing 10: 366–369
Brody S 1981 The concepts of attachment and bonding. Journal of American Psychoanalytic Association 29: 815–829
Butterfield P M, Emde R N, Svejda M J 1981 Does the early application of silver nitrate impair maternal attachment? Pediatrics 67: 737–738
Callaghan K 1979 Creating optimal environments for newborn infants and their families. Australian Nurses Journal 8: 14–16
Campbell S B, Taylor P M 1979 Bonding and attachment: theoretical issues. Seminars in Perinatology 3: 3–13
Carek D J, Capelli A J 1981 Mothers' reactions to their newborn infants. Journal of the American Academy of Child Psychiatry 20: 16–31
Carter-Jessop L 1981 Promoting maternal attachment through prenatal intervention. Maternal Child Nursing Journal 6: 107–112
Chang P N, Thompson T R, Fisch R O 1982 Factors affecting attachment between infants and mothers separated at birth. Journal of Developmental and Behavioral Pediatrics 3: 96–98
Chess S, Thomas A 1982 Infant bonding: mystique and reality. American Journal of Orthopsychiatry 52: 213–222
Cline F 1979 Lack of attachment in children. Nurse Practitioner 4: 35, 45
Craig S, Tyson J E, Samson J, Lasky R E 1982 The effect of early contact on maternal perception of infant behaviour. Early Human Development 6: 197–204
Cranley M S 1981 Roots of attachment: the relationship of parents with their unborn. Birth Defects 17: 59–83
Crockenberg S B 1981 Infant irritability, mother responsiveness, and social support influences on the security of mother-infant attachment. Child Development 52: 857–865
Dickerson P S 1981 Early postpartum separation and maternal attachment to twins. Journal of Obstetrics Gynecology and Neonatal Nursing 10: 120–123
Dunn D M, White D G 1981 Interactions of mothers with their newborns in the first half-hour of life. Journal of Advanced Nursing 6: 271–275
Egeland B, Sroufe L A 1981 Attachment and early maltreatment. Child Development

52: 44–52

Egeland B, Vaughn B 1981 Failure of 'bond formation' as a cause of abuse, neglect, and maltreatment. American Journal of Orthopsychiatry 51: 78–84

Gay J 1981 A conceptual framework of bonding. Journal of Obstetrics Gynecology and Neonatal Nursing 10: 440–444

Gordon A H, Jameson J C 1979 Infant-mother attachment in patients with non-organic failure to thrive syndrome. Journal of the American Academy of Child Psychiatry 18: 251–259

Gromada K 1981 Maternal-infant attachment: the first step toward individualizing twins. Maternal Child Nursing Journal 6: 129–134

Herbert M, Sluckin W, Sluckin A 1982 Mother-to-infant bonding. Journal of Child Psychology and Psychiatry 23: 205–221

Herbert P 1979 Rooming-in the newborn: getting to know baby — straight away. Nursing Mirror 149: 32–37

Holaday B 1981 Maternal response to their chronically ill infants' attachment behavior of crying. Nursing Research 30: 343–348

Hwang C P 1981 Aspects of the mother-infant relationship during nursing, 1 and 6 weeks after early extended post-partum contact. Early Human Development 5: 279–287

Klein R P, Durfee J T 1978 Effects of stress on attachment behavior in infants. Journal of Genetic Psychology 132 (second half): 321–322

Lamb M E 1979 Separation and reunion behaviors as criteria of attachment to mothers and fathers. Early Human Development 3: 329–339

Lamberg B R 1981 Eye opening of the newborn at and up to 20 minutes after birth. Journal of Advanced Nursing 6: 455–459

Lamperelli P, Smith J M 1979 The grieving process of adoption: an application of principles and techniques. Journal of Psychiatric Nursing 17: 24–29

Lederman R P, Lederman E, Work B A Jr, McCann D S 1979 Relationship of psychological factors in pregnancy to progress in labour. Nursing Research 28: 94–97

Mercer R T 1981 Factors impacting on the maternal role the first year of motherhood. Birth Defects 17: 233–252

Ogden T H 1979 On projective identification. International Journal of Psychoanalysis 60 (Pt 3): 357–373

Oseid B 1979 Breast-feeding and infant health. Seminars in Perinatology 3: 249–254

Paukert S 1982 Maternal-infant attachment in a traditional hospital setting. Journal of Obstetrics Gynecology and Neonatal Nursing 11: 23–26

Redshaw M, Rosenblatt D B 1982 The influence of analgesia in labour on the baby. Midwife Health Visitor Community Nurse 18: 126–132

Reiser S L 1981 A tool of facilitate mother-infant attachment. Journal of Obstetrics Gynecology and Neonatal Nursing 10: 294–297

Rhone M 1980 Six steps to better bonding. The Canadian Nurse 76: 38–41

Roberts J, Lynch M A, Golding J 1980 Postneonatal mortality in children from abusing families. British Medical Journal 281: 102–104

Ross G S 1980 Parental responses to infants in intensive care: the separation issue reevaluated. Clinics in Perinatology 7: 47–60

Siegel E 1982 Early and extended maternal-infant contact. A critical review. American Journal of Diseases of Children 136: 251–257

Svejda M J, Campos J J, Emde R N 1980 Mother-infant 'bonding': failure to generalize. Child Development 51: 775–779

Taylor L S 1981 Newborn feeding behaviors and attaching. Maternal Child Nursing 6: 201–202

Tracy R L, Ainsworth M D 1981 Maternal affectionate behavior and infant-mother attachment patterns. Child Development 52: 1341–1343

Tulman L J 1981 Theories of maternal attachment. Advances in Nursing Science 3:

7-14

Waters E, Vaughn B E, Egeland B R 1980 Individual differences in infant-mother attachment relationships at age one: antecedents in neonatal behavior in an urban, economically disadvantaged sample. Child Development 51: 208–216

Wise S, Grossman F K 1980 Adolescent mothers and their infants: psychological factors in early attachment and interaction. American Journal of Orthopsychiatry 50: 454–468

Whittlestone W G 1978 The physiology of early attachment in mammals: implications for human obstetric care. Medical Journal of Australia 1: 50–53

Adolescent pregnancy

In the last decade a rise in adolescent pregnancies has resulted in concern among care-providers, as this group has been shown to be at-risk both physically and psychologically in pregnancy. The authors represented in this section provide an overview of the major areas of concern related to adolescent pregnancy. The psychosocial research on causes of adolescent pregnancy and identification of adolescents at risk in the population is presented. There is information on family relations and potential modes of intervention; the short-and long-term prognosis for pregnancy in adolescents; the short-and long-term prognosis for the infant; the common complications of pregnancy; and the desirable services for pregnant adolescents and their families. A group of authors is also included who examine the interaction of adolescent development and the conflict this causes with becoming a parent during the teen years.

Baldwin W 1981 Adolescent pregnancy and childbearing: an overview. Seminars in Perinatology 5: 1–8

Baldwin W, Cain V S 1980 The children of teenage parents. Family Planning Perspectives 12: 34–39, 42–43

Billing-Meyer J 1979 A healthy child, a sure future. The single mother: can we help? The Canadian Nurse 75: 26–28

Bolton F 1980 The pregnant adolescent: problems of premature parenthood. Sage Publications, Beverly Hills

Brown H, Adams R G, Kellman S G 1982 A longitudinal study of teenage motherhood and symptoms of distress: The Woodlawn community epidemiological project. In: Simmons R (ed) Research in community and mental health, vol. 2. Journal of American International Press, Greenwich

Bryan-Logan B, Dancy B 1974 Unwed pregnant adolescents. Nursing Clinics of North America 9: 57–68

Campbell A 1968 The role of family planning in the reduction of poverty. Journal of Marriage and the Family 30: 236–246

Campbell B, Barnlund D 1977 Communication patterns and problems of pregnancy. American Journal of Orthopsychiatry 47: 134–139

Cannon-Bonventre K, Kahn J 1979 Interviews with adolescent parents. Children Today 8: 17–17

Carey W B, McCann-Sanford T, Davidson E C Jr 1981 Adolescent age and obstetric risk. Seminars in Perinatology 5: 9–17

Chelman C 1979 Adolescent sexuality in a changing American society. U.S.

Department of Health, Education and Welfare. Public Health Service Publication 79–1426

Coblinson W G 1981 Prevention of adolescent pregnancy: a developmental perspective. Birth Defects 17: 35–47

Coddington D R 1979 Life events associated with adolescent pregnancies. Journal of Clinical Psychology 40: 180–185

Colletta N D, Gregg C H 1981 How adolescents cope with the problems of early motherhood. Adolescence 16: 499–512

Cooper J C 1978 Pregnancy in adolescents: helping the patient and her family. Postgraduate Medicine 64: 60–64

Crabba P 1978 Social and emotional aspects of pregnancy in teenagers. Journal of Biosocial Sciences 5: 171–184

Daniels M B, Manning D 1983 A clinic for pregnant teens. American Journal of Nursing 83: 68–71

DeAmicis L A, Klotnon R, Hess D W, McQuarney E R 1981 A comparison of unwed teenagers and multigravid sexually active adolescents seeking contraception. Adolescence 16: 11–20

Donlen J, Lynch P 1981 Teenage mother: high risk baby. Nursing (Horsham) 1981 11: 51–56

Duenholler J H, Farog M D, Jiminez J M, Bouman G 1975 Pregnancy performance of patients under fifteen years of age. Obstetrics and Gynecology 46: 49–52

Elster A B, McQuarney E R 1980 Medical and psychological risks of pregnancy and childbearing during adolescence. Pediatric Annual 9: 89–94

Enos H M 1979 Goal setting with pregnant teenagers. Child Welfare 58: 541–542

Everett M 1980 Group work in the prenatal clinic. Health and Social Work 5: 71–74

Fisher S M, Scharf K R 1980 Teenage pregnancy: an anthropological sociological and psychological overview. Adolescent Psychiatry 8: 393–403

Fredman S B, Phillips S 1981 Psychological risk to mother and child as a consequence of adolescent pregnancy. Seminars in Perinatology 5: 33–37

Gabbard G D, Wolff J R 1977 The unwed pregnant teenager and her male relationships. Journal of Reproductive Medicine 19: 137–140

Hatcher S L 1976 Understanding adolescent pregnancy and abortion. Primary Care 3: 407–425

Hertz D G 1977 Psychological implications of adolescent pregnancy: patterns of family interaction in adolescent mothers to be. Psychosomatics 17: 13–16

Kandell N 1979 The unwed adolescent pregnancy: an accident? American Journal of Nursing 12: 2112–2114

Kinard E M, Kleinman L V 1980 Teenage parenting and child abuse: are they related? American Journal of Orthopsychiatry 50: 481–488

Klein L 1978 Antecedents of teenage pregnancy. Clinical Obstetrics and Gynecology 21: 1151–1159

Klerman L V 1980 Adolescent pregnancy: a new look at a continuing problem. American Journal of Public Health 70: 776–778

Laurence R A, Merritt T A 1981 Infants of adolescent mothers: perinatal, neonatal and infancy outcomes. Seminars in Perinatology 5: 19–32

Levenson P, Atkinson B, Hale J, Hollier M 1978 Adolescent parent education: a maturational model. Child Psychiatry and Human Development 9: 104–118

Mercer R T 1979 The adolescent parent, perspectives on adolescent health care. Lippincott, Philadelphia

Mercer R T 1980 Teenage motherhood: the first year. Journal of Obstetrics Gynecology and Neonatal Nursing 9: 16–27

Olson L 1980 Social and psychological correlates of pregnancy resolution among adolescent women: a review. American Journal of Orthopsychiatry 50: 432–455

Oppel W, Rayston A B 1971 Teen-age births: some social, psychological and physical sequelae. American Journal of Public Health 61: 751–756

Osofsky J D, Osofsky H J 1978 Teenage pregnancy: psychological considerations.

Clinical Obstetrics 21: 1161–1173

Panzarine S, Elster A, McQuarney E R 1981 Principles and practice: a systems approach to adolescent pregnancy. Journal of Obstetrics Gynecology and Neonatal Nursing 10: 287–289

Phipps-Yonas S 1980 Teenage pregnancy and motherhood: a review of the literature. American Journal of Orthopsychiatry 50: 403–410

Piersar E C 1978 Gynecologic approach to counselling the sexually active young woman. Clinics of Obstetrics and Gynecology 21: 235–239

Polley M J 1979 Teen mothers: a status report. Journal of School Health 49: 466–469

Robliss R 1981 A study of the relationship between adolescent pregnancy and life-change events. Issues in Mental Health Nursing 3: 219–236

Rosen R H 1980 Adolescent pregnancy decision making: are parents important? Adolescence 15: 43–54

Ruszala J 1980 Adolescent pregnancy. Nurse Practices 5: 22–24

Schwartz D D 1980 Perspectives on adolescent pregnancy. Wisconsin Medical Journal 79: 35–36

Steinhauf B 1979 Problem solving skills, locus of control and contraceptive effectiveness of young women. Child Development 50: 268–271

Tyrer L B, Mazler R G, Bradshaw L E 1978 Meeting the special needs of pregnant teenagers. Clinical Obstetrics and Gynecology 21: 1198–1213

Wilson F 1980 Antecedents of adolescent pregnancy. Journal of Biosocial Science 12: 141–152

Wise S, Grossman F 1980 Adolescent mothers and their infants: psychological factors in early attachment and interaction. American Journal of Orthopsychiatry 50: 454–468

Zongker C 1977 The self concept of pregnant adolescent girls. Adolescence 72: 477–488

Sexually transmitted diseases

With the increased frequency of premarital sexual activity, concern is being expressed regarding the increased risk of sexually transmitted diseases in pregnancy. This concern extends beyond the traditional venereal diseases of syphilis and gonorrhea to chlamydia and herpes infections. Left untreated, these diseases can give rise to fetal anomalies, fetal stillbirth and serious morbidity or early mortality in the newborn. The articles in this section were selected in order to provide an overview of the current incidence, identification and treatment of sexually transmitted diseases. The problems created by teenage intercourse are identified. There was little in the literature that related to appropriate modes of nursing intervention either in the area of casefinding or follow-up care, but the problem was seen to be of sufficient importance that it has been included. It is of particular importance to both public health nurses and those in occupational health where teaching can add to primary prevention.

Adler M N, Belsey E M, Rogers J S 1981 Sexually transmitted diseases in a defined population of women. British Medical Journal (Clinical Research) 283(6283): 29–32

Alexander E R 1979 Chlamydia: the organism and neonatal infection. Hospital Practice 14: 63–69

Alexander H 1982 Herpes simplex virus: a cause for concern. American Journal of
Medical Technology 48: 241–245
Campbell C E, Herten R J 1981 VD to STD: redefining venereal disease. American
Journal of Nursing 81(9): 1629–1635
Carbonetto C 1978 Neonatal gonococcal orogastric contamination. Journal of the
American Medical Association 249–861
Charles D 1980 Infections in obstetrics and gynecology. Major Problems in Obstetrics
and Gynecology 12: 1–427
Csonka G W, Coufalik E D 1977 Chlamydial, gonococcal, and herpes virus infections
in neonates. Postgraduate Medical Journal 53: 592–594
Cutler J C 1981 Venereal disease prevention. Cutis 27: 323–327
Diener B 1981 Cesarian section complicated by gonococcal ophthalmia neonatorum.
Journal of Family Practice 13: 739, 743–744
Doyle K L, Cassell C 1981 Teenage sexuality: the early adolescent years. Obstetrics
Gynecology Annual 10: 423–446
Duff P 1979 An evaluation of routine screening for gonorrhea in a population of
military dependents. Military Medicine 144(5): 322–325
Edwards L E, Barrada M I, Hamann A A, Hakanson E Y 1978 Gonorrhea in
pregnancy. American Journal of Obstetrics and Gynecology 132: 637–641
Edwards L E, Steinman M E, Hakanson E Y 1977 An experimental comprehensive
high school clinic. American Journal of Public Health 67: 765–766
Edwards M S 1978 Venereal herpes: a nursing overview. Journal of Obstetrics
Gynecology and Neonatal Nursing 7: 7–15
Eschenbach D A 1977 Sexually transmitted diseases: recent developments. In:
Castelazo-Ayala L et al (eds) Gynecology and obstetrics. Excerpta Medica,
Amsterdam, W3 EX89 no. 412, p 195–203
Eschenbach D 1977 Significance for the fetus of sexually acquired maternal infection
with mycoplasma, chlamydia, and Neisseria gonorrhoeae. Seminars in Perinatology
1: 11–24
Felman Y M 1979 A plea for the condom, especially for teenagers. Journal of the
American Medical Association 241: 2517–2518
Felman Y 1982 How useful are the serologic tests for syphilis? International Journal
of Dermatology 21: 79–81
Felman Y M 1978 Should premarital syphilis serologies continue to be mandated by
law? Journal of the American Medical Association 240: 459–460
Felman Y M, Nikitas J A 1981 Cytomegalovirus infection. Cutis 27: 562, 567–568,
570 passim
Goh T H, Ngeow Y F, Teoh S K 1981 Screening for gonorrhea in a prenatal clinic in
Southeast Asia. Sexually Transmitted Diseases 8: 67–69
Goodrich J T 1979 Treatment of gonorrhea in pregnancy. Sexually Transmitted
Diseases 6 (2 Suppl): 168–173
Grossman J 3rd 1977 Congenital syphilis. Teratology 16: 217–219
Gumpel J, Mejia 1978 Prenatal management, labour and delivery care and
postpartum follow-up of the drug addict. Journal of Reproductive Medicine 20:
333–336
Harris J K 1977 Human sexuality: implications for occupational health nursing.
Occupational Health Nursing (NY) 25: 7–10
Hinds M W 1977 Gonorrhea screening in family planning clinics when should it
become selective? Public Health Reports 92: 361–364
Huffman J W 1978 Gonorrhea: unmasking asymptomatic or atypical infection.
Postgraduate Medicine 63: 205–207
Jha P K, Singh G, Kaur P, Sharma D 1978 Unsuspected gonococcal infection in
female patients. British Journal of Venereal Disease 54: 324–325
Jones J E, Harris R E 1979 Diagnostic evaluation of syphilis during pregnancy.
Obstetrics and Gynecology 54: 611–614

Kampmeier R H 1981 The introduction of penicillin for the treatment of syphilis. Sexually Transmitted Diseases 8: 260–265

Kampmeier R H, Sweeney A, Quinn R W, Lefkowitz L B, Dupont W D 1981 A survey of 251 patients with acute syphilis treated in the collaborative penicillin study of 1943–1950. Sexually Transmitted Diseases 8: 266–279

Kraus S J 1979 Incidence and therapy of gonococcal pharyngitis. Sexually Transmitted Diseases 6 (2 Suppl): 143–147

Lossick J G 1979 Prevention and management of neonatal gonorrhea. Sexually Transmitted Diseases 6 (2 Suppl): 192–194

Lumicao G G, Heggie A D 1979 Chlamydial infections. Pediatric Clinics of North America 26: 269–282

Lutz B 1982 Gonococcal infections: new methods of treatment. Comprehensive Therapy 8: 47–52

Malvern J 1979 Perinatal infections: the obstetrician's viewpoint. CIBA Foundation Symposium (77): 215–227

McCormack W M 1979 Genital infections of perinatal importance. Clinics in Obstetrics and Gynecology 22: 313–319

McCormack W M 1982 Sexually transmitted diseases: women as victims (editorial). Journal of the American Medical Association 248: 177–178

McCormack W M, Nowroozi K, Alpert S, Sackel S G, Lee Y H, Lowe E W, Rankin J S 1977 Acute pelvic inflammatory disease: characteristics of patients with gonococcal and nongonococcal infection and evaluation of their response to treatment with aqueous procaine penicillin G and spectinomycin hydrochloride. Sexually Transmitted Diseases 4: 125–131

McNab W L 1979 The 'other' venereal diseases: herpes simplex, trichomoniasis and candidiasis. Journal of School Health 49: 79–83

Maw R D, Horner T 1981 Don't forget syphilis. Ulster Medical Journal 50: 132–136

Meissner J E 1979 Treating genital herpes. Nursing (Horsham) 9(7): 56–57

Mehta A, Wright T A 1977 Gonococcal arthritis in pregnancy. Canadian Medical Association Journal 117: 1190–1191

Morton R S, Gollow M M 1978 Laboratory support in the management of syphilis. Medical Journal of Australia 1: 378–383

Muir D G, Belsey M A 1980 Pelvic inflammatory disease and its consequences in the developing world. American Journal of Obstetrics and Gynecology 138 (7 Pt 2): 913–928

Newest treatment schedules for gonorrhoea. 1979 Medical Times 107: 15d–19d

Nunneley J B 1980 Special problems in women. Practitioner 224: 1145–1149

Oill P A, Mishell D R Jr 1980 Symposium on adolescent gynecology and endocrinology. Part III: Venereal diseases in adolescents and contraception in teenagers. Western Journal of Medicine 132: 39–48

Oppenheimer E H, Dahms B B 1981 Congenital syphilis in the fetus and neonate. Perspectives in Pediatric Pathology 6: 115–138

Oppenheimer E H, Winn K J 1981 Fetal gonorrhea with deep tissue infection occurring in utero. Pediatrics 69: 74–76

Oster H A 1981 Obstetric infections. Western Journal of Medicine 134: 394–404

Panconesi E, Zuccati G, Cantini A 1981 Treatment of syphilis: a short critical review. Sexually Transmitted Diseases 8 (4 suppl): 321–325

Phoon W O 1980 The implications on behavioral patterns of health and social changes. Tropical Doctor 10: 32–37

Plavidal F J, Werch A 1977 Gonococcal fetal scalp abscess: a case report. American Journal of Obstetrics and Gynecology 127: 437–438

Podgore J K, Holmes K K 1981 Ocular gonococcal infection with minimal or no inflammatory response. Journal of the American Medical Association 246: 242–243

Rees A, Tait I A, Hobson D, Byng R E, Johnson F W 1977 Neonatal conjunctivitis caused by Neisseria gonorrhoeae and Chlamydia trachomatis. British Journal of

Venereal Diseases 53: 173–179

Ridley C M 1980 Skin disorders of the vulva. Practitioner 224 (1343): 481–486

Rome R M 1978 Routine antenatal tests. Australian Family Physician 7: 1098–1103

Rothenberg R 1979 Ophthalmia neonatorum due to neisseria gonorrhoeae: prevention and treatment. Sexually Transmitted Diseases 6 (2 suppl): 187–191

Rozenbaum H 1978 Teenagers and contraception. International Journal of Gynaecology and Obstetrics 16: 564–567

Rudolph A H 1979 Antibiotic treatment of the venereal diseases — update 1979. International Journal of Dermatology 18: 797–804

Schneider G T 1979 Sexually transmissible vaginal infections in pregnancy. 1. Common infections. Postgraduate Medicine 65: 177–180

Schneider G T 1979 Sexually transmissible vaginal infections in pregnancy. 2. Less common infections. Postgraduate Medicine 65: 185–188

Schwarz R H, Crombleholme W R 1979 Antibiotics in pregnancy. Southern Medical Journal 72: 1315–1318

Seneca H 1982 Chlamydial infections. Comprehensive Therapy 8: 19–25

Shen J T 1982 Adolescent sexual behaviour. Postgraduate Medicine 71: 46–48, 50–51, 54–55

Smith J P 1979 The challenge of health education for nurses in the 1980s. Journal of Advanced Nursing 4: 531–543

Sparling P F 1979 Current problems in sexually transmitted diseases. Advances in Internal Medicine 24: 203–228

Spence M R 1977 Genital infections in pregnancy. Medical Clinics of North America 61: 139–151

Stark A R, Glode M P 1979 Gonococcal vaginitis in a neonate. Journal of Pediatrics 94: 298–299

Strand C L, Arango V A 1979 Gonococcal ophthalmia neonatorum after delivery by cesarian section: report of a case. Sexually Transmitted Diseases 6: 77–78

Taylor-Robinson D, McCormack W M 1980 The genital mycoplasmas (first of two parts). New England Medical Journal 302: 1003–1010

Treponemal infections. 1982 WHO Technical Report Service 674: 1–75

van der Lugt B, Drogendijk A C, Banffer J R 1980 Prevalence of cervical gonorrhoea in women with unwanted pregnancies. British Journal of Venereal Diseases 56: 148–150

Wager G P, Martin D H, Koutsky L, Eschenbach D A, Daling J R, Chiang W T, Alexander E R, Holmes K K 1980 Puerperal infectious morbidity: relationship to route of delivery and to antepartum Chlamydia trachomatis infection. American Journal of Obstetrics and Gynecology 138 (7 Pt 2): 1028–1033

Weinstein A J 1979 Treatment of bacterial infections in pregnancy. Drugs 17: 56–65

Westrom L 1980 Incidence, prevalence, and trends of acute pelvic inflammatory disease and its consequences in industrialized countries. American Journal of Obstetrics and Gynecology 138 (7 Pt 2): 880–892

Wilchins S 1978 Hemophilus vaginalis vaginitis and gonorrhea in pregnancy. Journal of Medical Sociology 75: 461–462

Willcox R R 1977 How suitable are available pharmaceuticals for the treatment of sexually transmitted diseases? (2) Conditions presenting as sores or tumours. British Journal of Venereal Diseases 53: 340–347

Fetal alcohol syndrome

Since the 1960s fetal teratogenesis has become of increasing concern to professionals in the field of maternal newborn care. Amongst the teratogens the role of alcohol in producing fetal anomalies is becoming increasingly recognized. A series of anomalies, including both physical symptoms and mental retardation, have become recognized as 'fetal alcohol syndrome'. The series of articles presented in this section cover the etiology of fetal alcohol syndrome; a review of the incidence of alcoholism in pregnancy; the relationship of maternal alcohol ingestion in pregnancy to the incidence of fetal/newborn symptoms; the common anomalies found in the fetus; suggested preventive measures; and finally evaluation and follow-up of women and infants who have been involved in preventive programs. It is hoped that the topics included will increase the nurse's knowledge of the disease and provide her with an effective knowledge base for working with women where alcoholism is either a diagnosed or potential problem.

Abel E H 1982 Characteristics of mothers of fetal alcohol syndrome children. Neurobehavioural Toxicology and Teratology 4: 3–4

Abel E H 1980 Fetal alcohol syndrome: behavioral teratology. Psychological Bulletin 87: 29–50

Alcohol and your unborn baby. 1980 AARN Newsletter 36: 1–2

Allen L H 1982 Calcium bioavailability and absorption: a review. American Journal of Clinical Nutrition 35: 783–808

Alpert J J, Day N, Dooling E, Hingson R, Oppenheimer E, Rosett H L, Weiner L, Zuckerman B 1981 Maternal alcohol consumption and newborn assessment: methodology of the Boston City Hospital prospective study. Neurobehavioural Toxicology and Teratology 3: 195–201

Altman G B 1980 Educational strategies for a community program in preventing alcohol use during pregnancy. Nursing Administration Quarterly 4: 23–29

Anderson R A Jr 1981 Endocrine balance as a factor in the etiology of the fetal alcohol syndrome. Neurobehavioural Toxicology and Teratology 3: 89–104

Arena J M 1979 Drug and chemical effects on mother and child. Pediatric Annals 8: 690–697

Ashley M J 1981 Alcohol use during pregnancy: a challenge for the 80s. Canadian Medical Association Journal 125: 141–143

Baghurst K I 1980 Nutritional and health aspects of alcohol consumption. Medical Journal of Australia 2: 177–178, 180

Beagle W S 1981 Fetal alcohol syndrome: a review. Journal of the American Dietetics Association 79: 274–276

Beattie J 1981 Fetal alcohol syndrome — the incurable hangover. Health Visitor 54: 468–469

Berkowitz G S 1981 An epidemiological study of preterm delivery. American Journal of Epidemiology 113: 81–92

Biggs J S 1981 Recognition of the 'at risk' pregnancy. Australian Family Physician 11: 71–75

Blomberg S 1980 Influence of maternal distress during pregnancy on fetal malformations. Acta Psychiatrica Scandinavia 62: 315–330

Blume S B 1981 Drinking and pregnancy: preventing fetal alcohol syndrome. New York State Journal of Medicine 81: 95–98

Bock J 1979 Closeup of fetal alcohol syndrome. The Canadian Nurse 75: 35

Bonnie R J 1980 Regulation of alcohol, tobacco, and other drugs: the agenda for law reform. National Institute Drug Abuse Research Monograph Series (34): 272–286

Cater J I 1980 Correlates of low birth weight. Child Care Health Deviation 6: 267–277

Chernoff G F 1979 Introduction: a teratologist's view of the fetal alcohol syndrome. Currents in Alcoholism 7: 7–13

Collins E 1980 Alcohol in pregnancy (editorial). Medical Journal of Australia 2: 173–175

Davidson F 1981 Smoking and alcohol consumption: advice given by health care professionals. Journal of Obstetrics Gynecology and Neonatal Nursing 10: 256–258

Davidson F, Alden L, Davidson P 1981 Changes in alcohol consumption after childbirth. Journal of Advanced Nursing 6: 195–198

Dening F C 1981 Alcohol and the unborn child. Midwives Chronicle 94: 196

Dolan M 1979 Alcoholism: the all-American addiction. American Pharmaceutics 19: 26–29

Dowdell P M 1981 Alcohol and pregnancy: a review of the literature 1968–1980. Nursing Times 77: 1825–1831

Drinks anyone? 1981 Australian Family Physician 10: 939

Dunigan T H, Werlin S L 1981 Extrahepatic biliary atresia and renal anomalies in fetal alcohol syndrome. American Journal of Diseases of Children 135: 1067–1068

Edmondson H A 1980 Pathology of alcoholism. American Journal of Clinical Pathology 74: 725–742

Erb L, Andresen B D 1981 Hyperactivity: a possible consequence of maternal alcohol consumption. Pediatric Nursing 7: 30–33, 51

Eriksson M, Larsson G, Zetterstrom R 1979 Abuse of alcohol, drugs and tobacco during pregnancy — consequences for the child. Paediatrician 8: 228–242

Evans A N, Brooke O G, West R J 1980 The ingestion by pregnant women of substances toxic to the fetus. Practitioner 224: 315–319

Fetal-alcohol syndrome. 1979 Paediatric Annals 8: 119–120

Finnegan L P 1981 The effects of narcotics and alcohol on pregnancy and the newborn. Annals of the New York Academy of Science 362: 136–157

Fisher S E, Atkinson M, Burnap J K, Jacobson S, Sehgal P K, Scott W, Van Thiel D H 1982 Ethanol-associated selective fetal malnutrition: a contributing factor in the fetal alcohol syndrome. Alcoholism (NY) 6: 197–201

Fitzsimons R B, Mahoney M J, Cussen G H 1981 Ethanol intoxication of the newborn: a case report and review of the literature. Irish Medical Journal 74: 230–231

Friedman J M 1982 Can maternal alcohol ingestion cause neural tube defects? Journal of Paediatrics 101: 232–234

Froede R C, Gordon J D 1980 Alcoholism — the second greatest imitator. An introduction to the problem of alcoholism. American Journal of Clinical Pathology 74: 719–720

Gaerlan M 1980 Understanding the physiology of alcohol abuse. The Canadian Nurse 76: 46–49

Gaines J 1981 The right to quality life: a challenge for parenting education. Health Education (Washington) 12: 18–20

Harlap S, Shiono P H 1980 Alcohol, smoking, and incidence of spontaneous abortions in the first and second trimester. Lancet 2(1817): 173–176

Heine M W 1981 Alcoholism and reproduction. Progress in Biochemical Pharmacology 18: 75–82

Henderson G I, Patwardhan R V, Hoyumpa A M Jr, Schenker S 1981 Fetal alcohol syndrome: overview of pathogenesis. Neurobehavioural Toxicology and Teratology 3: 73–80

Horrobin D F 1980 A biochemical basis for alcoholism and alcohol-induced damage including the fetal alcohol syndrome and cirrhosis: interference with essential fatty acid and prostaglandin metabolism. Medical Hypotheses 6: 929–942

Johnson K G 1979 Fetal alcohol syndrome: rhinorrhea, persistent otitis media, choanal stenosis, hypoplastic sphenoids and ethmoid. Rocky Mountain Meddical Journal 76: 64–65

Kaminski M, Franc M, Lebouvier M, du Mazaubrun C, Rumeau-Rouquette C 1981 Moderate alcohol use and pregnancy outcome. Neurobehavioural Toxicology and Teratology 3: 173–181

Kessler D B. Newberger E H 1981 At risk: the developing infant. Child Today 10: 10–14

Kline J, Shrout P, Stein Z, Susser M, Warburton D 1980 Drinking during pregnany and spontaneous abortion. Lancet 2(8187): 176–180

Krous H F 1981 Fetal alcohol syndrome: a dilemma of maternal alcoholism. Pathology Annual 16 (Pt 1): 295–311

Kuzma J W, Kissinger D G 1981 Patterns of alcohol and cigarette use in pregnancy. Neurobehavioural Toxicology and Teratology 3: 211–212

Lillien L J, Hubre A M, Rajala M M 1982 Diet and ethanol intake during pregnancy. Journal of the American Dietary Association 81: 252–257

Little R E 1980 Maternal alcohol and tobacco use and nausea and vomiting during pregnancy: relation to infant birthweight. Acta Obstetrica Gynecologica Scandinavia 59: 495–497

Little R E, Grathwohl H L, Streissguth A P, McIntyre C 1981 Public awareness and knowledge about the risks of drinking during pregnancy in Multnomah County, Oregon. American Journal of Public Health 71: 312–314

Little R E, Hook E B 1979 Maternal alcohol and tobacco consumption and their association with nausea and vomiting during pregnancy. Acta Obstetrica Gynecologica Scandinavia 58: 15–17

Little R E Streissguth A P, Barr II M, Herman C S 1980 Decreased birth weight in prevention. Canadian Medical Association Journal 125: 159–164

Little R E streissguth A P, Barr H M, Herman C S 1980 Decreased birth weight in infants of alcoholic women who abstained during pregnancy. Journal of Pediatrics 96: 974–977

Little R E, Streissguth A P, Guzinski G M 1980 Prevention of fetal alcohol syndrome: a model program. Alcoholism (NY) 4: 185–189

Mau G 1980 Moderate alcohol consumption during pregnancy and child development. European Journal of Paediatrics 133: 233–237

McMillen M 1980 Alcohol education: fetal alcohol syndrome. Oklahoma Nurse 25: 5

Meeting special needs. 1980 Nursing Administration Quarterly 4: 61–74

Minor M J, Van Dort D 1982 Prevention research on the teratogenic effects of alcoholics. Currents in Alcoholism 8: 301–314

Morrisey E R 1981 The stress of children's births: gender differences in the impact on alcoholics. Current in Alcoholism 8: 301–314

Morrison A B, Maykut M O 1979 Potential adverse effects of maternal alcohol ingestion on the developing fetus and their sequelae in the infant and child. Canadian Medical Association Journal 120: 826–828

Newman N M, Correy J F 1980 Effects of alcohol in pregnancy. Medical Journal of Australia 2: 5–10

Olegard R, Saebl K G, Aronsson M, Sandin B Johansson P R, Carlsson C, Kyllerman M, Iversen K, Hrbek A 1979 Effects on the child of alcohol abuse during pregnancy. Retrospective and prospective studies. Acta Obstetrica Gynecologica Scandinavia [Suppl] 275: 112–121

Pelosi M A, Langer A, Apuzzio J, Kaminetzky H A, Fricchione D 1980 Drinking and pregnancy. Journal of the Medical Society of New York 77: 101–102

Pierog S, Chandavasu O, Wexler I 1979 The fetal alcohol syndrome: some maternal characteristics. International Journal of Gynaecology and Obstetrics 16: 412–415

Powell J J 1981 The tragedy of fetal alcohol syndrome. RN 81 44: 33–35, 92–96

Pratt O E 1981 Alcohol and the developing fetus. British Medical Bulletin 38: 48–52

Rayburn W F, Motley M E, Zuspan F P 1982 Conditions affecting nonstress test results. Obstetrics and Gynecology 59: 490–493

Reading A E, Campbell S, Cox D N, Sledmere C M 1982 Health beliefs and health care behaviour in pregnancy. Psychological Medicine 12: 379–383

Reiff J S 1980 Fetal alcohol syndrome. Maryland State Medical Journal 29: 20–21

Rivard C 1979 The fetal alcohol syndrome. Journal of School Health 49: 96–98

Robe L B, Gromisch D S, Iosub S 1981 Symptoms of neonatal ethanol withdrawal. Currents in Alcoholism 8: 485–493

Rohner S W 1980 Fetal alcohol effects linked to moderate drinking levels. Maryland State Medical Journal 29: 26–27

Rosenlicht J, Murphy J B, Maloney P L 1979 Fetal alcohol syndrome. Oral Surgery 47: 8–10

Rosett H L 1980 A clinical perspective of the Fetal Alcohol Syndrome. Alcoholism (NY) 4: 119–122

Rosett H L, Weiner L 1981 Identifying and treating pregnant patients at risk from alcohol. Canadian Medical Association Journal 125: 149–154

Rosett H L, Weiner 1981 Prevention of fetal alcohol effects. Pediatrics 69: 813–816

Rosett H L, Weiner L, Edelin K C 1981 Strategies for prevention of fetal alcohol effects. Obstetrics and Gynecology 57: 1–7

Rosett H L, Weiner L, Zuckerman B, McKinlay S, Edelin K C 1980 Reduction of alcohol consumption during pregnancy with benefits to the newborn. Alcoholism (NY) 4: 178–184

Russell M, Bigler L 1979 Screening for alcohol-related problems in an outpatient obstetric-gynecologic clinic. American Journal of Obstetrics and Gynecology 134: 4–12

Sardor G G, Smith D F, MacLeod P M 1981 Cardiac malformations in the fetal alcohol syndrome. Journal of Pediatrics 98: 771–773

Small W E 1979 Warning — alcohol may be hazardous to your baby. American Pharmaceutics 19: 16–17

Smith D W 1980 Alcohol effects on the fetus. Progress in Clinical Biological Research 36: 73–82

Smith D W 1981 Fetal alcohol syndrome and fetal alcohol effects. Neurobehavioural Toxicology and Teratology 3: 127

Smith D W 1979 The fetal alcohol syndrome. Hospital Practice 14: 121–128

Smith I E 1979 Fetal alcohol syndrome: a review. Journal of the Medical Association of Georgia 68: 799–804

Smith J P 1979 The challenge of health education for nurses in the 1980s. Journal of Advanced Nursing 4: 531–543

Smith R 1981 Alcohol, women, and the young: the same old problem? British Medical Journal [Clinical Research] 283: 1170–1172

Sokol R J 1981 Alcohol and abnormal outcomes of pregnancy. Canadian Medical Association Journal 125: 143–148

Sokol R J, Miller S I, Reed G 1980 Alcohol abuse during pregnancy: an epidemiological study. Alcoholism (NY) 4: 135–145

Spiegel P G, Pekman W M, Rich B H, Versteeg C N, Nelson V, Dudnikov M 1979 The orthopedic aspects of the fetal alcohol syndrome. Clinical Orthopedics 139: 58–63

Steeg C N, Woolf P 1979 Cardiovascular malformations in the fetal alcohol syndrome. American Heart Journal 98: 635–637

Stephens C J 1981 The fetal alcohol syndrome: cause for concern. Maternal Child Nursing Journal 6: 251–256

Streissguth A P, Barr H M, Martin D C, Herman C S 1980 Effects of maternal alcohol, nicotine, and caffeine use during pregnancy on infant mental and motor development at eight months. Alcoholism (NY) 4: 152–164

Streissguth A P, Martin D C, Martin J C, Barr H M 1981 The Seattle longitudinal prospective study on alcohol and pregnancy. Neurobehavioural Toxicology and Teratology 3: 223–233

Surgeon general's advisory on alcohol and pregnancy. 1981 Food and Drug Administration Bulletin 11: 9–10

Tennes K, Blackard C 1980 Maternal alcohol consumption, birth weight, and minor physical anomalies. American Journal of Obstetrics and Gynecology 138 (7 Pt 1): 774–780

Teschke R, Rauen J, Neufeind M, Petrides A S, Strohmeyer G 1980 Alcoholic liver disease associated with increased gamm-glutamyltransferase activities in serum and liver. Advances in Experiments in Medical Biology 132: 647–654

Thadani P V 1981 Fetal alcohol syndrome: neurochemical and endocrinological abnormalities. Progress in Biochemical Pharmacology 18: 83–98

Thompson M A 1980 Alcohol and pregnancy — part 2: Studies in man. Food and Cosmetic Toxicology 18: 314–316

Toutant C, Lippmann S 1980 Fetal alcohol syndrome. American Family Physician 22: 113–117

Umbreit J, Ostrow L S 1980 The fetal alcohol syndrome. Mental Retardation 18: 109–111

van den Berg B J 1981 Maternal variables affecting fetal growth. American Journal of Clinical Nutrition 34 (Suppl 4): 722–726

Walpole I R, Hockey A 1980 Fetal alcohol syndrome: implications to family and society in Australia. Australian Pediatric Journal 16: 101–105

Weathersbee P S, Lodge J R 1979 Alcohol, caffeine, and nicotine as factors in pregnancy. Postgraduate Medicine 66: 165–167, 170–171

Weiner L, Rosett H L, Edelin K C 1982 Behavioral evaluation of fetal alcohol education for physicians. Alcoholism (NY) 6: 230–233

Williams B 1979 The effect of maternal alcohol consumption during pregnancy. Journal of the Medical Association of Georgia 68: 805–809

Wilson J 1981 The fetal alcohol syndrome. Public Health 95: 129–132

Wilson M 1981 Fetal alcohol syndrome — the American scene. Nursing Times 77: 1832–1835

Wright J M 1981 Fetal alcohol syndrome: the social work connection. Health and Social Work 6: 5–10

Woolf P 1979 Maternal alcohol ingestion and pregnancy. Midwife Health Visitor Community Nurse 15: 308–310

Woollam D H 1981 Alcohol and the safety of the unborn child. Social Health Journal 101: 241–244

Genetic counselling

Since the advent of the electron microscope geneticists have achieved major advances in recognizing a variety of chromosomal and genetically transmitted anomalies. As a result, genetic counselling has become available for parents where there is a potential risk for an abnormal fetus. Nurses are becoming involved in genetic screening and in supportive care and follow-up of parents who select termination of pregnancy when a fetal anomaly is diagnosed. The authors in this section have been selected in order to provide an overview of the whole counselling field. Attention is paid to the overall principles of counselling; preparation of the counselors; the role of the counselor; risk factors in specific conditions; tests and procedures that follow counselling; and evaluation and follow-up of parents who have received genetic counselling. Specific tools for history taking, such as a genetic family history questionnaire, are described within these readings. The nurse's role in relation to counselling and to specific procedures, such as amniocentesis, is described. Many of the articles emphasize that the counselor's role is to provide information so that parents can make informed choices. Some of the evaluative studies that are reported question the parents' understanding of information that has been provided. For any nurse interested in the field of genetic counselling these readings should provide a balanced view of the current strengths and weaknesses of the professional's ability to help parents who seek genetic information.

Abramovsky I, Godmilow L, Hirschorn K, Smith H Jr 1980 Analysis of a follow-up study of genetic counselling. Clinics in Genetics 17: 1–12

Adler R 1979 It doesn't end with death. Clinical Pediatrics 18: 767–768

Anderson L, Cowan B 1982 The expanded role of the pregnancy counselor. Family and Community Health 5: 13–18

Auntley R M 1979 Genetic counselling: problems of sociological research in evaluating the quality of counselor decision making. American Journal of Medical Genetics 4: 1–4

Bartai I, Vullo C 1980 Assessment of prospective genetic counselling in the Ferarra area. American Journal of Medical Genetics 6: 195–204

Bochkov N P, Kozlova S I 1978 Evaluation of genetic consultations in the public health service. Human Genetics 41: 189–195

Braitman A, Auntley R M 1978 Development of instruments to measure counselor's knowledge of Down's syndrome. Clinical Genetics 13: 25–36

Carter C O 1978 Genetic counselling. British Journal of Hospital Medicine 19: 557–562

Cole J P, Conneally P M, Hodes M E, Merritt A D 1978 Genetic family history questionnaire. Journal of Medical Genetics 15: 10–19

Connor A F 1977 Congenital malformations and genetic counselling. Medical Journal of Australia 1: 805–807

Curran W J 1978 Genetic counselling and wrongful life. American Journal of Public Health 68: 501–502

Creizel A, Metneki J, Oszlovics M 1980 Evaluation of information-guidance genetic counselling. Journal of Medical Genetics 18: 91–98

Davies B L, Doran T A 1981 Factors in a woman's decision to undergo genetic amniocentesis for advanced maternal age. Nursing Research 31: 56–59

Dicker M, Dicker L 1978 Genetic counselling as an occupational specialty: a sociological perspective. Social Biology 25: 272–278

Emery A H, Raeburn J A, Skinner R, Holloway S, Lewis P 1979 Prospective study of genetic counselling. British Medical Journal 1: 1253–1256

Fielding J E, Russo P K 1978 Genetic counselling for the older pregnant woman: new data and questions. Massachusetts Department of Public Health 298: 1419–1421

Finley S 1978 Genetic counselling. Pediatric Annals 7: 19–24

Finley W H 1978 Delivering genetic services. Pediatric Annals 7: 13–16

Genetic Counselling 1979 The National Foundation, March of Dimes Box 2000 White Plains, New York

Haseltine F P 1981 Genetic approach to gynecologic and obstetrics problems. Primary Care 8: 89–110

Headings V E 1975 Genetic counselling models for genetic disorders. Social Biology 22: 297–303

Hockey A, Michael C A, Bain J G 1979 Genetic screening in Western Australia. Medical Journal of Australia 1: 363–365

Hogan R, Tcheng D 1978 The role of the nurse during amniocentesis. Journal of

Obstetrics Gynecology and Neonatal Nursing 7: 24–27

Hook E B 1979 Genetic counselling dilemmas: Downs Syndrome, paternal age and recurrence risk after remarriage. American Journal of Medical Genetics 5: 145–151

Jackson L G 1976 Prenatal genetic counselling. Primary Care 3: 701–716

Juberg R C 1978 Fetal and maternal indications for considering abortion. Southern Medical Journal 71: 50–57

Kessler S 1980 Genetic associates/counsellors in genetic services. American Journal of Medical Genetics 7: 323–334

Kessler S 1981 Psychological aspects of genetic counselling: analysis of a transcript. American Journal of Medical Genetics 8: 137–153

Leonard C O, Chase G A, Childs B 1972 Genetic counselling: a consumer view. New England Journal of Medicine 287: 433–439

Lippman-Hand A, Fraser F C 1979 Genetic counselling: provision and reception of information. American Journal of Medical Genetics 3: 113–127

Lippman-Hand A, Fraser F C 1979 Genetic counselling: the postcounselling period 1. Parents perceptions of uncertainty. American Journal of Medical Genetics 4: 51–71

Malter S 1977 Genetic counselling ... a responsiblity of health care professionals. Nursing Forum 16: 27–35

McCormack M K 1979 Medical genetics and family practice. Practical Therapeutics 20: 143–154

McDonough P G 1978 Antenatal diagnosis. Postgraduate Medicine 63: 161–167

Naylor E W 1975 Genetic screening and genetic counselling: knowledge, attitudes and practices in two groups of family planning professionals. Social Biology 22: 304–314

Nitowsky H M 1976 Genetic counselling: objectives, principles and procedures. Clinical Obstetrics and Gynaecology 19: 919–940

Pauker S P, Pauker S G 1977 Prenatal diagnosis: a directive approach to genetic counselling using decision analysis. The Yale Journal of Biology and Medicine 50: 275–289

Polani P E, Alberman E, Alexander B J, Benson P F, Berry A C et al 1979 Sixteen years' experience of counselling, diagnosis, and prenatal detection in one genetic centre: progress, results and problems. Journal of Medical Genetics 16: 166–175

Passarge E 1980 The delivery of genetic counselling services in Europe. Human Genetics 56: 1–5

Riccardi V M 1976 Health care and disease prevention through genetic counselling: a regional approach. American Journal of Public Health 66: 268–272

Riccardi V M, Cohen A, Chen M T 1978 Genetic counselling as part of hospital care. American Journal of Public Health 68: 652–655

Scrimgeout J B 1978 Genetics: antenatal diagnosis in early pregnancy. British Journal of Hospital Medicine 19: 565–573

Seldenfeld M J, Antley R M 1981 Genetic counselling: a comparison of counselee's genetic knowledge before and after (Part III). American Journal of Medical Genetics 10: 107–112

Shanklin E, Kenen R 1979 Foretelling the genetic future. Ethics in Science and Medicine 6: 21–30

Simpson N E, Dallaire L, Miller J R, Simonovich L, Hamerton J L, Miller J, McRikeen C 1976 Prenatal diagnosis of genetic disease in Canada: report of a collaborative study. Canadian Medical Journal 23: 739–745

Simpson J L, Elias S, Gatlin M, Martin A O 1981 Genetic counselling and genetic services in obstetrics and gynecology: implications for educational goals and clinical practice. American Journal of Obstetrics and Gynecology 140: 70–80

Tishler C L 1981 The psychological aspects of genetic counselling. American Journal of Nursing 81: 733–734

Tsuang M T 1978 Genetic counselling for psychiatric patients and their families. American Journal of Psychiatry 135: 1465–1475

Weiss J O 1976 Social work and genetic counselling. Social Work in Health Care 2: 5–12

Wright E E 1980 The legal implications of refusing to provide prenatal diagnosis in low-risk pregnancies solely for sex selection. American Journal of Medical Genetics 5: 391–397

Management of pain in labour

A great deal of controversy exists on the long-term effects of medication given in labour on the newborn. Parents express anxiety about medication given to the mother inhibiting maternal-newborn bonding. Preparation for childbirth is seen as a means of reducing maternal anxiety and tension and thus decreasing pain perception in labour and thus the need for medication in labour. Articles in this section provide an overview of the physiological and psychological components of pain. The role of childbirth preparation is presented and critiqued. Methods of pain relief are presented and evaluated, including one of the newer techniques, transcutaneous nerve stimulation. The role of the nurse in pain relief with some potentially useful nursing activities are discussed. The effect of medication on the newborn is evaluated in two studies presented in this section.

Beck N C, Siegel L J 1980 Preparation for childbirth and contemporary research on pain, anxiety and stress reduction: a review and critique. Psychosomatic Medicine 42: 429–447

Beck N C, Siegel L J, Davidson N P, Kormeier S, Breitenstein A, Hall D G 1980 The prediction of pregnancy outcome: maternal preparation, anxiety and attitudinal sets. Journal of Psychosomatic Research 24: 343–351

Blackwell J 1978 Labour pains. Nursing Mirror 146: 28–29

Brown C 1982 Therapeutic effects of bathing during labour. Journal Nurse Midwifery 27: 13–16

Bundsen P, Peterson L E, Selstam U 1981 Pain relief in labour by transcutaneous electrical nerve stimulation. A prospective matched study. Acta Obstetrica Gynecologica Scandinavia 60: 459–468

Bundsen P, Ericson K 1982 Pain relief in labor by transcutaneous electrical nerve stimulation. Safety aspects. Acta Obstetrica Gynecologica Scandinavia 61: 1–5

Bundsen P, Ericson K, Peterson L E, Thiringer K 1982 Pain relief in labour by transcutaneous electrical nerve stimulation. Testing of a modified stimulation technique and evaluation of the neurological and biochemical condition of the newborn infant. Acta Obstetrica Gynecologica Scandinavia 61: 129–136

Connolly A M, Pancheri P, Lucchetti A, Salmaggi L, Guerrieri D, Francalancia M, Bartoleschi A, Zichella L 1978 Labour as a psychosomatic condition: a study of the influence of personality on self-reported anxiety and pain. In: Carenza L et al (eds) Clinical psychoneuroendocrinology in reproduction. Academic Press, London, 22: 369–379

Davies J M, Rosen M 1977 Intramuscular diazepam in labour. A double-blind trial in multiparae. British Journal Anaesthesia 49: 601–604

Erkkola R, Pikkola P, Kanto J 1980 Transcutaneous nerve stimulation for pain relief during labour: a controlled study. Annales Chirurgiae et Gynaecologiae 69: 273–277

Fishburne J I 1982 Systematic analgesia during labor. Clinical Perinatology 9: 29–53

Genest M 1981 Preparation for childbirth — evidence for efficacy. A review. Journal of Obstetrics Gynaecology and Neonatal Nursing 10: 82–85

Gitsch E, Kubista E 1980 [The influence of transcerebral impulse current on labour pain and the course of delivery (author's transl)] Geburtshilfe und Fraunheilkunde 40: 406–411

Hodgkinson R, Husain F J 1982 The duration of effect of maternally administered meperidine on neonatal neurobehaviour. Anesthesiology 56: 51–52

Kitzinger S 1978 Pain in childbirth. Journal of Medical Ethics 4: 119–121

Lanahan C C 1978 Variables affecting pain perception during labor. Current Practices in Obstetrical and Gynecological Nursing 2: 149–156

Marinova M, Smilov I 1980 [Transcutaneous electrical nerve stimulation (TENS) in obstetrical practice (a review of the literature)] Akusherstvo Ginekologiia (Sofiia) 19: 366–373

Marshall K 1981 Pain relief in labor. The role of the physiotherapist. Physiotherapy 67: 8–11

Melzack R, Taenzer P, Feldman P, Kinch R A 1981 Labor is still painful after prepared childbirth training. Canadian Medical Association Journal 125: 357–363

Morgan B, Bulpitt C J, Clifton P, Lewis P J 1982 Effectiveness of pain relief in labor: survey of 100 mothers. British Medical Journal (Clinical Research) 285: 689–690

Mozingo J N 1978 Pain in labour: a conceptual model for intervention. Journal of Obstetrics Gynecology and Neonatal Nursing 7: 47–49

Nel C P, Bloch B, Rush J M 1981 A comparison of meptazinol and pethidine for pain relief during the first stage of labour. South African Medical Journal 59: 908–910

Nesheim B I 1981 The use of transcutaneous nerve stimulation for pain relief during labor. A controlled clinical study. Acta Obstetrica Gynaecologica Scandinavia 60: 13–16

Norr K L, Block C R, Charles A, Meyering S, Meyers E 1977 Explaining pain and enjoyment in childbirth. Journal of Health and Social Behaviour 18: 260–275

Nursing management of pain. A study of comfort measures during labor. 1977 Nursing Journal of India 68: 259–260

Ounsted M, Simons C 1979 Maternal attitudes to their obstetric care. Early Human Development 3: 201–204

Roberts J, Malasanos L, Mendez-Bauer C 1981 Maternal positions in labor: analysis in relation to comfort and efficiency. Birth Defects 17: 97–128

Roberts J E 1983 Factors influencing distress from pain during labour. American Journal of Maternal Child Nursing 8: 62–66

Robinson J O, Rosen M, Evans J M, Revill S I, David H, Rees G A 1980 Self-administered intravenous and intramuscular pethidine. A controlled trial in labour. Anaesthesia 35: 763–770

Scambler A 1979 New standards in childbirth control. Midwife Health Visitor Community Nurse 15: 449–450

Scott-Palmer J, Skevington S M 1981 Pain during childbirth and menstruation: a study of locus control. Journal of Psychosomatic Research 25: 151–155

Silverstone A C 1981 Recent changes in labor management. Nursing (Horsham) 21: 924–926

Vadurro J F, Butts P A 1982 Reducing the anxiety and pain of childbirth through hypnosis. American Journal of Nursing 82: 620–623

Worthington E L Jr, Martin G A 1980 A laboratory analysis of response to pain after training with three Lamaze techniques. Journal of Psychosomatic Research 24: 109–116

Wright J T 1981 Abnormal labor and pain relief. Nursing (Horsham) 21: 921–923

Care of the mother with a Cesarian section

With the increasing rate of Cesarian sections in modern hospitals, concern has been expressed about the effects of surgery on maternal well-being. The evidence suggests that unanticipated surgery creates feelings of inadequacy regarding the individual woman's success as a mother. There also seems to be some indication that maternal-newborn bonding is less effective. In this section of the bibliography articles have been selected that focus on the psychological consequences of Cesarian section. The articles range from reports of mothers regarding their own feelings following section to the presentation of research on mothers' post-section. Nursing intervention helpful to mothers following surgery are described. Some initial problems with mother-infant bonding, particularly following anesthetic, are described. Reading the articles in this section will increase the nurse's understanding of the needs of the mother following an unanticipated Cesarian section and should enhance her ability to provide appropriate nursing care.

Affonso D D 1981 Parent infant acquaintance: interacting variables when birth is a cesarian. In Affonso D (ed) Impact of a Cesarian birth. Davis, Philadelphia.

Affonso D D, Stichler F F 1980 Cesarian birth women's reactions. American Journal cesarian birth. Birth and the Family Journal 5: 88–94

Affonso D D, Stichler F F 1980 cesarian birth women's reactions. American Journal of Nursing 80: 468–470

Affonso D D, Stichler F F 1981 Impact on women: Feelings and perceptions. In: Affonso D (ed) Impact of Cesarian birth. Davis, Philadelphia

Bampton B, Mancine J 1973 The cesarian section patient is a new mother too. Journal of Obstetrics Gynecology and Neonatal Nursing 2: 58–61

Birdsong L S 1981 Loss and grieving in cesarian mothers. In: C F Kehoe (ed) The Cesarian birth experience. Appleton-Century-Crofts, New York

Cohen N W 1977 Minimizing emotional sequelae of cesarian childbirth. Birth and the Family Journal 4: 114–119

Conklin M M 1977 Discussion groups for cesarian section. Journal of Obstetrics Gynecology and Neonatal Nursing 6: 52–54

Corner B S 1977 Teaching about cesarian birth in traditional childbirth classes. Birth and the Family Journal 4: 107–113

Donovan B 1977 The Cesarian birth experience. Beacon Press, Boston

Donovan B, Allen R M 1977 The cesarian birth method. Journal of Obstetrics Gynecology and Neonatal Nursing 6: 37–38

Enkin M 1977 Having a section is having a baby. Birth and the Family Journal 4: 99–101

Evrard J R, Gold E M 1978 Cesarian section: risk/benefit. Perinatal Care 2: 4–10

Frantz K B 1979 Breast feeding works for cesarian sections too... and here is precisely how you can help the mother do it. RN 42: 38–47

Gunn C 1967 Cesarian section. Nursing Times 63: 425–426

Harris J K 1980 Symposium on the selfcare concept of nursing. Self care is possible after cesarian delivery. Nursing Clinics of North America 15: 191–204

Hart G 1980 Maternal attitudes in prepared and unprepared cesarean deliveries. Journal of Obstetrics Gynecology and Neonatal Nursing 9: 243–245

Hedahl K J 1980 Cesarian birth: a real family affair. American Journal of Nursing 80: 471–472

Hedahl K J 1980 Working with families requiring a cesarian birth. Pediatric Nursing 6: 1–5

Kehoe C F 1981 Identifying the nursing needs of the postpartum cesarian mother. In: Kehoe C F (ed) The caesarian birth experience. Appleton-Century-Crofts, New York

Kehoe C F 1981 The cesarian birth experience. Appleton-Century-Crofits, New York

Lipson J G, Tilden V P 1980 Psychological integration of the cesarian birth experience. American Journal of Orthopsychiatry 50: 598–609

Marut J S 1978 The special needs of the cesarian mother. American Journal of Maternal Child Nursing 3: 202–206

Marut J S, Mercer R T 1979 Comparison of primiparas' perceptions of vaginal and cesarian births. Nursing Research 228: 260–266

Mercer R T, Marut J 1981 Comparative viewpoints: cesarian versus vaginal childbirth. In: Affonso D D (ed) Impact of Cesarian birth, Davis, Philadelphia

Mercer R T 1981 Potential effects of anesthesia and analgesia on the maternal-infant attachment process of cesarian mothers. In: Kehoe C E (ed) The cesarean birth experience, Appleton-Century-Crofts, New York

Mevs L 1977 The current status of cesarian section and today's maternity patient. Journal of Obstetrics Gynecology and Neonatal Nursing 6: 44–47

NIH Consensus Development Conference 1981. Cesarean childbirth. Clinical Pediatrics 20: 555–558

Placek P J, Vaffel S M 1980 Trends in cesarean section: rates for thee U.S. Public Health Reports 95: 540–548

Reynolds C B 1977 Cesarian section: Facts and Futures. Updating care of cesarean section patients. Journal of Obstetrics Gynecology and Neonatal Nursing 6: 48–51

Schlosser S 1978 The emergency cesarian section...why she needs help...what you can do. RN 41: 52–57

Stichler J F, Affonso D D 1980 Caesarian birth. American Journal of Nursing 80: 466–468

Stockamer C 1980 The myth and reality of Cesareans. Journal of Paediatric Nursing 30: 18–22

Stockamer C 1980 Cesarean patients: delivering the right kind of care. Journal of Practical Nursing 30: 17–18

Tryphmopoulou Y, Doxiadis S 1972 The effect of elective section on the initial stages of mother-infant relationships. In: Morris N (ed) Psychosomatic medicine in Obstetrics and Gynecology, S. Kargar, Basel

Wilson C C, Hovey W R 1980 Cesarean childbirth. New American Library, New York

Fathers and pregnancy

Societal changes have altered the father's role to one of closer involvement in childbearing and childrearing. Fathers today seek involvement in prenatal classes, in labour and delivery and recognize a need to bond with their child. The authors in this section discuss the psychological issues such as parental attachment to the fetus and newborn bonding. The fathers' own feelings related to their exclusion in matters relating to the development and birth of their child are reported. Nursing interventions which may be helpful to the father, and to the developing family, during the antepartum, labour and delivery and postpartum periods are included. Several articles relate to the father's presence at Cesarian sections. This section on fathers and pregnancy contains a comprehensive overview on the concerns of fathers and the ways in which their involvement in childbearing can be facilitated.

Annexton M 1978 Parent-infant bonding sought in 'birthing' centers. Journal of the American Medical Association 240: 823

Blackwell J 1977 Husband in the labour ward. Midwives Chronicle 90: 270–272

Bowen S M, Miller B C 1980 Paternal attachment behavior as related to presence at delivery and preparenthood classes: a pilot study. Nursing Research 29: 307–334

Boyd S T, Mahon P 1980 The family-centered caesarean delivery. Maternal Child Nursing Journal 5: 176–180

Boyd S, Stafford A 1976 Father involvement in cesarean section delivery. Texas Medicine 76: 54–55

Briggs E 1979 Transition to parenthood. Maternal Child Nursing Journal 8: 69–83

Brown H 1979 Fathers and childbirth: changing attitudes and expectations. Midwife Health Visitor Community Nurse 15: 398–400

Campbell A, Worthington E L Jr 1982 Teaching expectant fathers how to be better childbirth coaches. Maternal Child Nursing Journal 7: 28–32

Caparulo F, London K 1981 Adolescent fathers: adolescents' first, fathers second. Issues in Health Care of Women 3: 23–33

Clulow C, Cleavely E, Coussell P, Dearnley B 1979 Love's labour and loss. Health Visitor 52: 74–76

Collier P 1982 A practitioner comments on research findings. Understanding couvade. Maternal Child Nursing Journal 7: 114

Cranley M S 1981 Roots of attachment: the relationship of parents with their unborn. Birth Defects 17: 59–83

Davies M 1977 National Childbirth Trust: antenatal teaching. Nursing Times 73: 1646–1647

DeGarmo E 1978 Fathers' and mothers' feelings about sharing the childbirth experience. Current Practices in Obstetrical and Gynecological Nursing 2: 162–174

DeGarmo E, Davidson K 1978 Psychosocial effects of pregnancy on the mother, father, marriage, and family. Current Practices in Obstetrical and Gynaecological Nursing 2: 24–44

Dodendorf D M 1981 Expectant fatherhood and first pregnancy. Journal of Family Practice 13: 744–751

Fishbein E G 1981 Fatherhood and disturbances of mental health: a review. Journal of Psychiatric Nursing 19: 24–27

Fries M E 1977 Longitudinal study: prenatal period to parenthood. Journal of the American Psychoanalytic Association 25: 115–132

Gabel H 1982 Childbirth experiences of unprepared fathers. Journal of Nurse Midwifery 27: 5–8

Gerzi S, Berman E 1981 Emotional reactions of expectant fathers to their wives' first pregnancy. British Journal of Medical Psychology 54 (Pt 3): 259–265

Goldsach G 1979 Why my wife received no ante-natal care for six months: a father's view of pregnancy and childbirth. Health Visitor 52: 77–78

Gregory S 1981 The father's class. Nursing Times 77: 1894–1897

Handshin J S 1981 Perspectives on the father's childbearing role. Australian Nurses Journal 10: 50–52

Hangsleben K L 1980 Transition to fatherhood: literature review. Issues in Health Care of Women 2: 81–97

Hedahl K J 1980 Cesarean birth: a real family affair. American Journal of Nursing 80: 471–472

Heggenhougen H K 1980 Father and childbirth: an anthropological perspective. Journal of Nurse Midwifery 25: 21–26

Hutchins P 1979 New fathers. Midwife Health Visitor Community Nurse 15: 10–11

Hutchins P, Harvey D 1977 A supplement on parentcraft. 2. The father's role. Nursing Mirror 145: v–vi, xi

Jennings B, Edmundson M 1980 The postpartum period: after confinement: the fourth trimester. Clinical Obstetrics and Gynecology 23: 1093–1103

Kunst-Wilson W, Cronenwett L 1981 Nursing care for the emerging family: promoting paternal behavior. Research in Nursing and Health 4: 201–211

Lamb G S, Lipkin M Jr 1982 Somatic symptoms of expectant fathers. Maternal Child Nursing Journal 7: 110–113, 115

Leonard L 1977 The father's side; a different perspective on childbirth. The Canadian Nurse 73: 16–20

Leonard L, Wortherspoon L 1982 And father makes three... The Canadian Nurse 78: 38–41

May K A 1978 Active involvement of expectant fathers in pregnancy: some further considerations. Journal of Obstetrics Gynecology and Neonatal Nursing 7: 7–12

May K A 1980 A typology of detachment/involvement styles adopted during pregnancy by first-time expectant fathers. Western Journal of Nursing Research 2: 444–461

May K A 1982 The father as observer. Maternal Child Nursing Journal 7: 319–322

McKee L 1980 Fathers and childbirth: 'Just hold my hand.' Health Visitor 53: 368–372

McKenzie R A 1980 The road to fatherhood: one man's personal remembrances. Issues in Health Care of Women 2: 99–106

MacLaughlin S 1980 First-time fathers' childbirth experience. Journal of Nurse Midwifery 25: 17–21

McQuaid P E 1979 Occasional topic. The child is father of the man. Irish Journal of Medical Science 148: 329–334

Nadelson C C, Notman M T 1977 Treatment of the pregnant teenager and the putative father. Current Psychiatric Therapy 17: 81–88

Panzarine S, Elster A B 1982 Prospective adolescent fathers: stresses during pregnancy and implications for nursing interventions. Journal Psychosocial Nursing Mental Health Services 20: 21–24

Peterson G H, Mehl L E, Leiderman P H 1979 The role of some birth-related variables in father attachment. American Journal of Orthopsychiatry 49: 330–338

Pies H E 1978 The right of a father to be present in the delivery room. Journal of Nurse Midwifery 22: 46–47

Pomatto M C 1981 Concerns of fathers throughout the childbearing cycle: a review of the literature. Kansas Nurse 56: 16–17

Reynolds D 1979 Mum's the word for babies in hospital. Nursing Mirror 48: 20–22

Rodholm M, Larsson K 1979 Father-infant interaction at the first contact after delivery. Early Human Development 3: 21–27

Shannon-Babitz M 1979 Addressing the needs of fathers during labor and delivery. Maternal Child Nursing Journal 4: 378–382

Sprunger L W, Preece E W 1981 Characteristics of prenatal interviews provided by pediatricians. Clinics in Pediatrics (Phila) 20: 778–782

Stanton M E 1979 The myth of 'natural' childbirth. Journal Nurse Midwifery 24: 25–29

Swartz R 1977 A father's view. Children Today 6: 14–17

Taubenheim A M 1981 Paternal-infant bonding in the first-time father. Journal of Obstetrics Gynecology and Neonatal Nursing 10: 261–264

Thompson H 1982 Antenatal care: what about father? Community Outlook 14: 99–104

Valvanne L 1980 [Who is wanted in the delivery room?] Katilolehti 85: 200–202

Waletzky L R 1979 Husbands' problems with breast-feeding. American Journal of Orthopsychiatry 49: 349–352

Williamson P, English E C 1981 Stress and coping in first pregnancy: couple-family physician interaction. Journal of Family Practice 13: 629–635

Transport of the newborn

In areas of the world where geographical distance isolates rural families from easy access to centers able to care for the at-risk newborn, transport becomes a critical factor in relation to newborn survival. Prevention of oxygen deprivation, cold stress and subsequent hypoglycemia are critical factors in developing safe modes of transport. The literature in this section identifies the persistent problems inherent in the transport of the sick newborn in situations where the place of birth is distant from the specialized care institution. The desirability of transporting the mother is addressed. The need to stabilize the newborn prior to transport, modes of stabilization, prevention of hypoxia, hypothermia and hypoglycemia are included. The articles cover both research literature and articles describing the experience of neonatal teams in transport; personnel needed; and the required educational preparation for personnel. Long-term effects of separation of mother and newborn are described.

Anderson E, Pederson V F 1979 Transport of high risk newborn infants. Danish Medical Bulletin 26: 147–149

Anderson C L, Aladjem S, Ayerste O, Caldwell C, Ismail M 1981 An analysis of maternal transport within a suburban metropolitan region. American Journal of Obstetrics 140: 499–504

Babson S G, Benson R C, Pernoll M I 1975 Management of high risk pregnancy and intensive care of the neonate. Mosby, St Louis

Blake A M, McIntosh N, Reynolds E O R, Ondres G 1975 Transport of newborn infants for intensive care. British Medical Journal 4: 13–17

Boehm F H, Haire M F 1979 One way maternal transport: An evolving concept. American Journal of Obstetrics and Gynecology 134: 484–489

Boehm F H, Haire M F, Davidson K, Barnett D R, Killam R P 1979 Maternal-fetal transport: Inpatient and outpatient scores. Journal of Tennessee Medical Association 72: 829–833

Bowen P A 1980 Regional centers: Part II. The newborn transport system. Issues in Health Care of Women 5–6: 5–17

Brown F B 1978 The development of high-risk obstetric transfer patients. Obstetrics and Gynecology 81: 674–676

Capobianco J A 1980 Keeping the newborn warm: how to safeguard the infant against life-threatening heat loss. Nursing 80 10: 64–67

Chance G W, Mathew J D, Williams G 1978 Neonatal transport: a controlled study of skilled assistance. Journal of Pediatrics 93: 662–666

Chester M 1977 Air travel designed for premies ... neonatal transport service. Stanford University Medical Service, California. Life Health 92: 30–31

Clarke T A, Zmora E, Chen J H, Reddy G, Merritt T A 1980 Transcutaneous oxygen monitoring during neonatal transport. Pediatrics 65: 884–886

Cox N C 1980 The nurse's role in transporting the critically ill child. Current Practices in Pediatric Nursing 3: 240–266

Dahlenburg G W 1977 Transport of the critically ill newborn infant in South Australia. Australasia Nursing Journal 7: 37–41

Davis V 1980 The structure and function of brown adipose tissue in the neonate.

Journal of Obstetrics Gynecology and Neonatal Nursing 9: 368–372

Ciles H R, Isaman J, Moore J W, Christian L D 1977 The Arizona high-risk maternal transport system: an initial view. American Journal of Obstetrics and Gynecology 128: 400–407

Greene W T 1980 Organization of neonatal transport services in support of a regional referral center. Clinical Perinatology 7: 187–195

Gunn T, Outerbridge E W 1978 Effectiveness of neonatal transport. Canadian Medical Association Journal 118: 646–649

Guy M 1978 Symposium on neonatal care...Children's Hospital of Los Angeles: neonatal transport. Nursing Clinics of North America 13: 3–11

Haasis P, Goldsmith J P 1979 A prototype perinatal transport system. The EMT Journal 3: 46–51

Harris B A Jr, Wintschafer D D, Huddleston J F, Perlis H W 1981 In utero versus neonatal transportation of high risk perinates: a comparison. Obstetrics and Gynecology 57: 496–499

Hein H A, Erenberg A P, Lane N, Lundvall J 1978 Transport of the high risk neonate: who, when, and how. Journal of Iowa Medical Society 68: 348–357

Johnson P J, Jung A L, Boros S J 1979 Neonatal nurse practitioners: a new expanded nursing role II. Perinatology and Neonatology 3: 25

Johnson S H 1977 Data gathering tool: an interactional deprivation of mother and premature infant. Community Nursing Research 9: 102–110

Jones P K, Halliday H L, Jones S L 1979 Prediction of neonatal death on need for interhospital transfer by prenatal risk characteristics of mother. Medical Care 17: 796–806

Kisling J A, Schreiner R L 1977 Transport of critically ill neonates: a new role for respiratory therapists. Respiratory Therapy 7: 47–50

Klauss M, Fanaroff A A 1973 Care of the high risk neonate. Saunders, Philadelphia

Ledger W J 1980 Identification of the high risk mother and fetus...does it work? Clinical Perinatology 7: 125–134

Levy D L, Noelke K, Goldsmith J P 1981 Maternal and infant transport program in Louisiana. Obstetrics and Gynecology 57: 500–504

Merenstein G B, Pettet G, Woodall J, Hill J 1977 An analysis of air transport results in the sick newborn: antenatal and neonatal referrals. American Journal of Obstetrics and Gynecology 128: 520–525

Miller C, Clyman R I, Roth R S, Sniderman S H, Ballard R A, Herring D, Riedel P, Rosen A, Burden L 1980 Control of oxygenation during the transport of sick neonates. Pediatrics 66: 117–119

Modanlau H D, Dorchester W, Freeman R K, Rommal C 1980 Perinatal transport to a regional perinatal center in a metropolitan area: maternal versus neonatal transport. American Journal of Obstetrics and Gynecology 138: 1157–1164

Morris F Jr, Brumley G 1971 Evaluation of a new infant transport incubator in North Carolina. North Carolina Medical Journal 32: 383

Pearl K 1981 Neonatal transport the Canadian way. Midwife Health Visitor Community Nurse 17: 152–154

Perez R C, Burks R 1978 Transporting high risk infants. Journal of Emergency Nursing 4: 14–18

Ramamurthy R S, Yeh T F, Pildes R S 1976 Transport of high risk neonates Part II: short term intensive care and stabilization of the sick infant. Illinois Medical Journal 150: 601–604

Segal S 1972 Manual for the transport of high risk newborn infants: principles, policies, equipment, techniques. Canadian Pediatric Society, Sherbrooke

Shepard K 1970 Air transport of high-risk infants utilizing a flying intensive care nursery. Journal of Pediatrics 77: 148–149

Stevens D C, Schreiner R L 1980 Complications of parturition: potential benefits of prenatal transport. Indiana State Medical Association Journal 7: 474–475

Thompson T R 1980 Neonatal transport nurses: an analysis of their role in the
    transport of newborn infants. Pediatrics 65: 887–892
Tooley W H 1977 Neonatal transport: a discussion. Respiratory Care 22: 1138–1145
Usher R 1977 Changing mortality rates with perinatal intensive care and
    regionalization. Seminars in Perinatology 1: 309–319
Washington S 1978 Temperature control of the neonate. Nursing Clinics of North
    America 13: 23–28
Williams J K, Lancaster J 1976 Thermoregulation of the newborn. Maternal Child
    Nursing Journal 1: 355–360

Grief and grieving

The majority of articles in this section relate to grieving in relation to perinatal death. However, other aspects of grief related to infertility, abortion, unanticipated cesarian section and the birth of a child with a congenital anomaly are also included. The relationship of both nurse and physician to grieving families is critical to grief resolution and the writings of some authors concerned with this topic are included. A few articles that outline common causes of perinatal death are also included, as it is felt that knowledge in this area will enable the midwife or maternity nurse to provide better anticipatory guidance for parents.

Birtchnell J, Kennard J 1982 Some marital and child-rearing characteristics of early
    mother-bereaved women. British Journal of Medical Psychology 55 (Pt 2): 177–186
Bracey J 1981 Aftercare in mourning. Nursing Times 77: 282–283
Caplan G 1981 Mastery of stress: psychosocial aspects. American Journal of
    Psychiatry 138: 413–420
Chase T M 1980 Perinatal death: initiating positive family grief. Journal of the
    Medical Association of the State of Alabama 50: 26–27
Clyman R I, Green C, Mikkelsen C, Rowe J, Ataide L 1979 Do parents utilize
    physician follow-up after death of their newborn? Pediatrics 64: 665–667
Croucher M 1982 Stillbirth. Nursing Mirror 155(1): xv–xvi
Crout T K 1980 Caring for the mother of a stillborn baby. Nursing (Horsham) 10:
    70–73
Dunlop J L 1979 Bereavement reaction following stillbirth. Practitioner 222: 115–118
Elliott B A, Hein H A 1978 Neonatal death: reflections for physicians. Pediatrics 62:
    96–100
Foyn S, Hatlestad A 1980 [Birth of a physically handicapped child]. Sykepleien 67:
    6–11
Grace J T 1978 Good grief: coming to terms with the childbirth experience. Journal of
    Obstetrics Gynecology and Neonatal Nursing 7: 18–22
Harrington V 1982 Bereavement and childbirth: look, listen and support. Nursing
    Mirror 154: 21–28
Harvey K 1977 Caring perceptively for the relinquishing mother. Maternal Child
    Nursing Journal 2: 24–28
Kimbrough C A 1981 The review and grief work of a multipara upon birth of a live
    infant. Maternal Child Nursing Journal 10: 207–213
Kirkley-Best E, Kellner K R 1982 The forgotten grief: a review of the psychology of
    stillbirth. American Journal of Orthopsychiatry 52: 420–429
Knapp R J, Peppers L G 1979 Doctor-patient relationships in fetal/infant death

encounters. Journal of Medical Education 54: 775–780

Kowalski K 1980 Managing perinatal loss. Clinical Obstetrics and Gynecology 23: 1113–1123

Kowalski K, Osborn M R 1977 Helping mothers of stillborn infants to grieve. Maternal Child Nursing Journal 2: 29–32

Jolly H 1977 Loss of a baby. Australian Nurses Journal 7: 40–41

LaRoche C, Lalinec-Michaud M, Engelsmann F, Fuller N, Copp M, Vasilevsky K 1982 Grief reactions to perinatal death: an exploratory study. Psychosomatics 23: 510–511, 514, 516–518

Lewis E, Page A 1978 Failure to mourn a stillbirth: an overlooked catastrophe. British Journal of Medical Psychology 51: 237–241

Limerick L 1979 Counselling parents who have lost an infant. Journal of the Royal College of Physicians of London 13: 242–245

McCain C 1981 How to work more comfortably with grief: your own and your patients': we're never prepared for infant death. Nursing life 1: 52

Menning B E 1982 The psychosocial impact of infertility. Nursing Clinics of North America 17: 155–163

Mercer R T 1981 The nurse and maternal tasks of early postpartum. Maternal Child Nursing Journal 6: 341–345

Middleton J 1979 The perinatal bereavement crisis. Michele and James. Journal of Nurse Midwifery 24: 19–21

O'Donohue N 1979 The perinatal bereavement crisis. Facilitating the grief process. Journal of Nurse Midwifery 24: 16–19

Opirhory G J 1979 Counselling the parents of a critically ill newborn. Journal of Obstetrics Gynecology and Neonatal Nursing 8: 179–182

Parrish S 1980 Letting go. Canadian Nurse 76: 34–37

Phillips L 1981 The effects of perinatal death. Midwife Health Visitor Community Nurse 17: 18–21

Quirk T R 1979 The perinatal bereavement crisis. Crisis theory, grief theory, and related psychosocial factors: the framework for intervention. Journal of Nurse Midwifery 24: 13–16

Rowe J, Clyman R, Green C, Mikkelsen C, Haight J, Ataide L 1978 Follow-up of families who experience a perinatal death. Pediatrics 62: 166–170

Sahu S 1981 Coping with perinatal death. Journal of Reproductive Medicine 26: 129–132

Savage W 1978 Perinatal loss and the medical team. Part 1. Midwife Health Visitor Community Nurse 14: 292–295

Savage W 1978 Perinatal loss and the medical team. Part 2. Midwife Health Visitor Community Nurse 14: 348–351

Saylor D E 1977 Nursing response to mothers of stillborn infants. Journal of Obstetrics Gynecology and Neonatal Nursing 6: 39–42

Schlosser S 1978 The emergency C-section patient: why she needs help — what you can do. RN 1978 41: 52–57

Schodt C M 1982 Grief in adolescent mothers after an infant death. Image 14: 20–25

Shepard T H, Fantel A G 1979 Embryonic and early fetal loss. Clinical Perinatology 6: 219–243

Short R V 1978 When a conception fails to become a pregnancy. CIBA Foundation Symposium 64: 377–394

Speck P 1978 Easing the pain and grief of stillbirth. Nursing Mirror 146: 38–41

Stack J M 1980 Spontaneous abortion and grieving. American Family Physician 21: 99–102

Stubblefield P G, Berek J S 1980 Perinatal mortality in term and post-term births. Obstetrics and Gynecology 56: 676–682

Turco R 1981 The treatment of unresolved grief following loss of an infant. American Journal of Obstetrics and Gynecology 141: 503–507

Vines D 1979 Bonding, grief, and working through in relationship to the congenitally anomalous child and his family. American Nurses Association Publication (NP-59): 185–192

Worlow D 1978 What do you say when the baby is stillborn? RN 1978 41: 74

Yong R K 1977 Chronic sorrow: parent's response to the birth of a child with a defect. Maternal Child Nursing Journal 2: 38–42

Index

expressed breast milk and, 130–131, 142, 143
follow-up services, 137, 144
getting to know baby, 133–134
going home without baby, 133
at home, 136–137, 142
information giving, 131–132, 140, 143
   misunderstanding and, 140–141
   written information, 141–142
mothers' needs, 131–134
mothers' reactions to baby, 128–129
need for stimulation, 136, 141
parents support group, 137

photographs of babies, 132, 142, 143, 144
telephone enquiries, 132–133, 144
timing of first NICU visit, 127–128
visiting, 132–133, 134, 142, 143
see also Low birthweight infant

Wrongful birth, 5–6
Wrongful life, 5